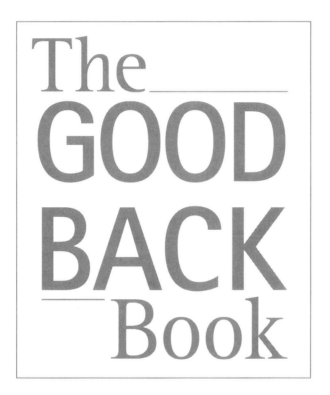

The
GOOD
BACK
Book

Renita Fehrsen-Du Toit

FIREFLY BOOKS

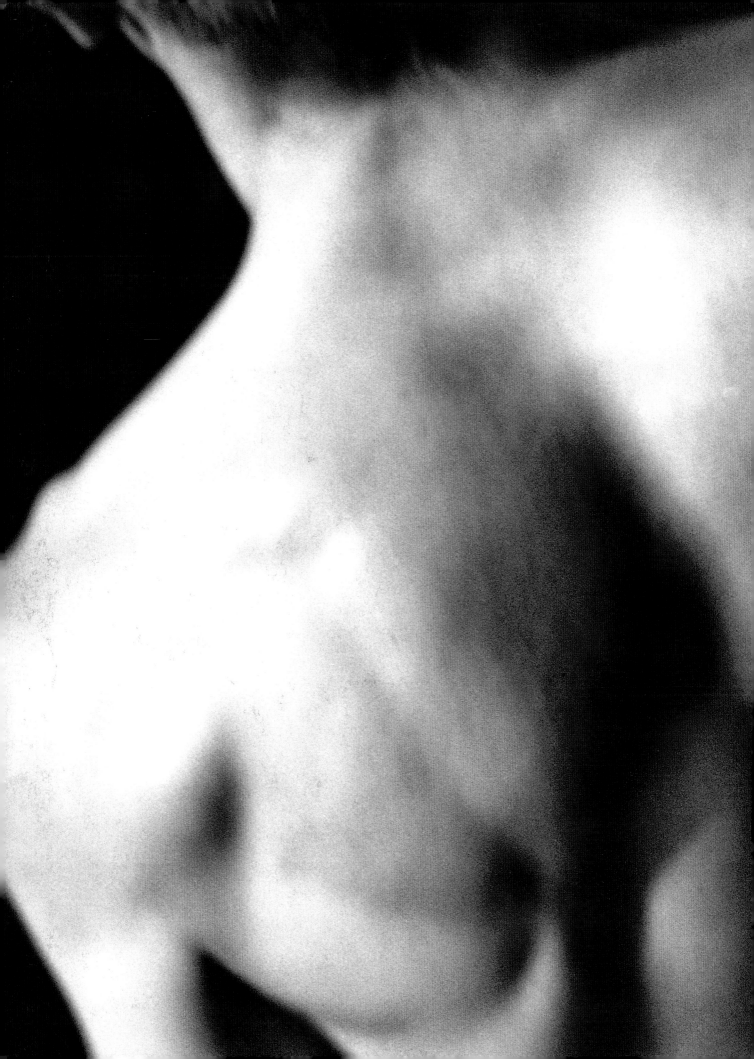

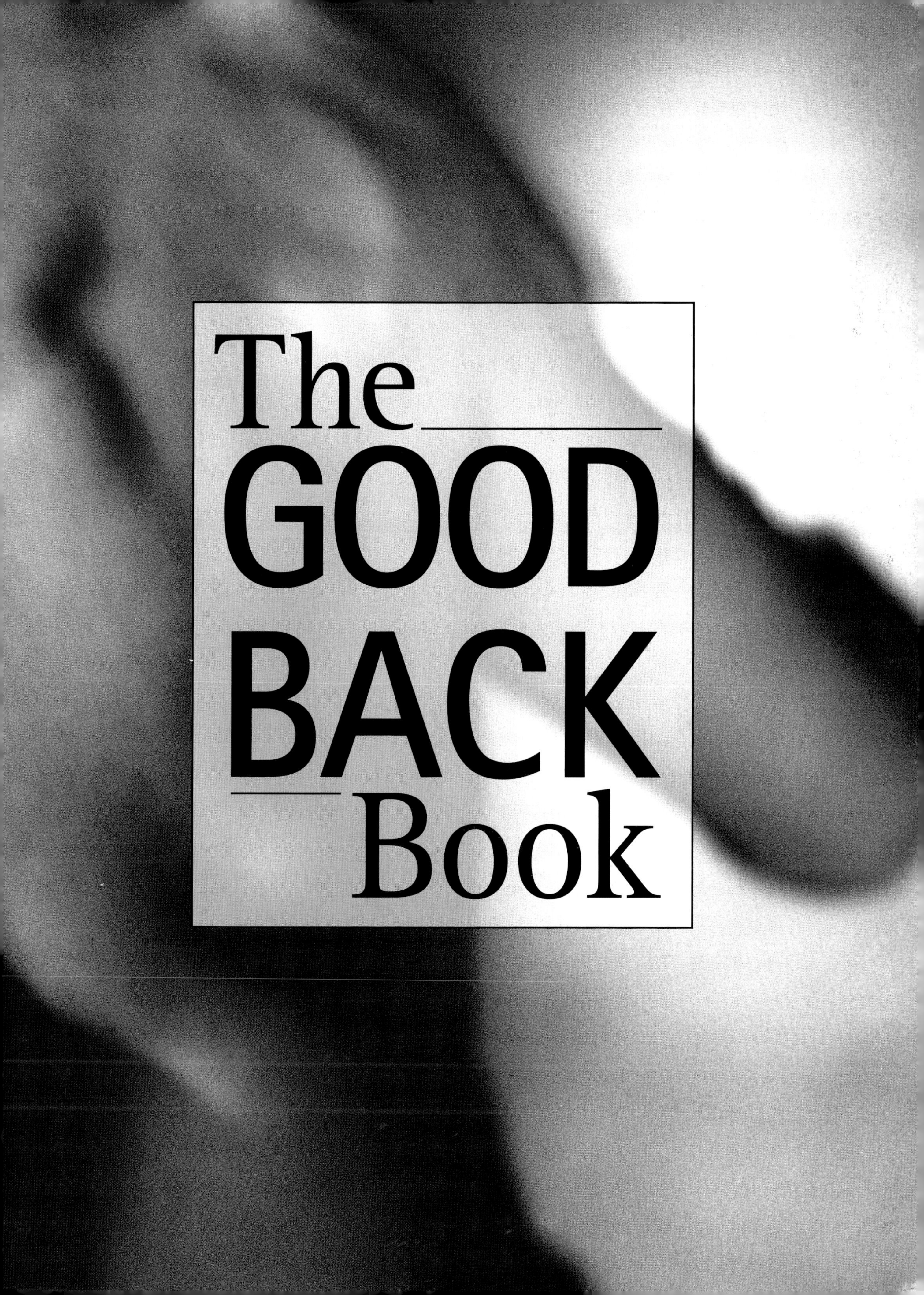

The GOOD BACK Book

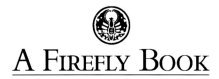

A FIREFLY BOOK

Published by Firefly Books Ltd., 2003
Copyright © 2002 New Holland Publishers (UK) Ltd

First Printing

National Library of Canada Cataloguing in Publication Data

Fehrsen-Du Toit, Renita
  The good back book: a practical guide to alleviating and preventing back pain / Renita Fehrsen-Du Toit. – 1st North American ed.
Includes index
ISBN 1-55297-827-3 (bound). – ISBN 1-55297-826-5 (pbk.)
1. Backache – Prevention. 2. Backache – Treatment. 3. Back – Care and hygiene. 1. Title
RD768.F47 2003   617.5'6   C2003-0900393-0

Publisher Cataloging-in-Publication Data (U.S.)

Toit, Renita Fehrsen-Du.
The good back book : a practical guide to alleviating and preventing back pain /
Renita Fehrsen-Du Toit. — 1st American ed.
[128] p. ; col. ill. , photos. : cm.
Includes index.
Summary: Guidance on understanding spine anatomy and how common back problems occur, how to improve posture, how strengthen the back and prevent problems, and detailed instructions on useful exercises.
ISBN 1-55297-827-3
ISBN 1-55297-826-5 (pbk.)
1. Backache — Exercise therapy. 2. Backache — Prevention. I. Title.
617.5/ 64062 21 RD771.B217.T6462 2003

First published in Canada in 2003 by
Firefly Books Ltd.
3680 Victoria Park Avenue
Toronto, Ontario M2H 3K1

First Published in the United States in 2003 by
Firefly Books (U.S.) Inc.
P.O. Box 1338, Ellicott Station
Buffalo, New York 14205

PUBLISHER Mariëlle Rensen
PUBLISHING MANAGERS Claudia dos Santos & Simon Pooley
MANAGING ART EDITOR Richard MacArthur
COMMISSIONING EDITOR Karyn Richards
EDITOR Ingrid Corbett
DESIGNER Geraldine Cupido
PICTURE RESEARCH Karla Kik and Bronwyn Allies
ILLUSTRATOR Steven Felmore
PRODUCTION Myrna Collins
CONSULTANT Dr. Ian Drysdale, Principal, British College of Osteopathic Medicine
Reproduction by Hirt & Carter (Cape) Pty Ltd
Printed and bound in Malaysia by Times Offset (M) Sdn Bhd

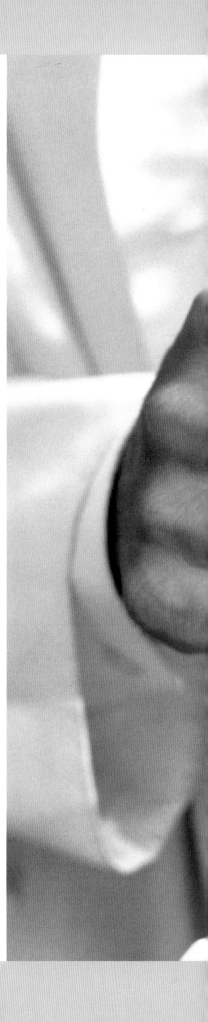

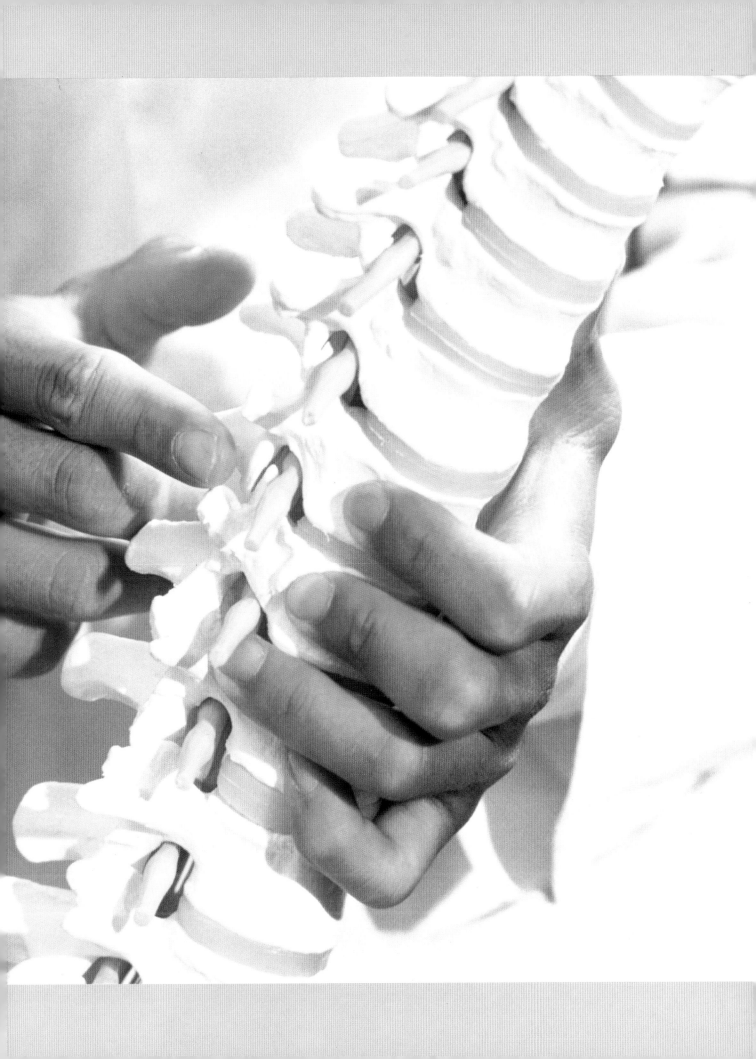

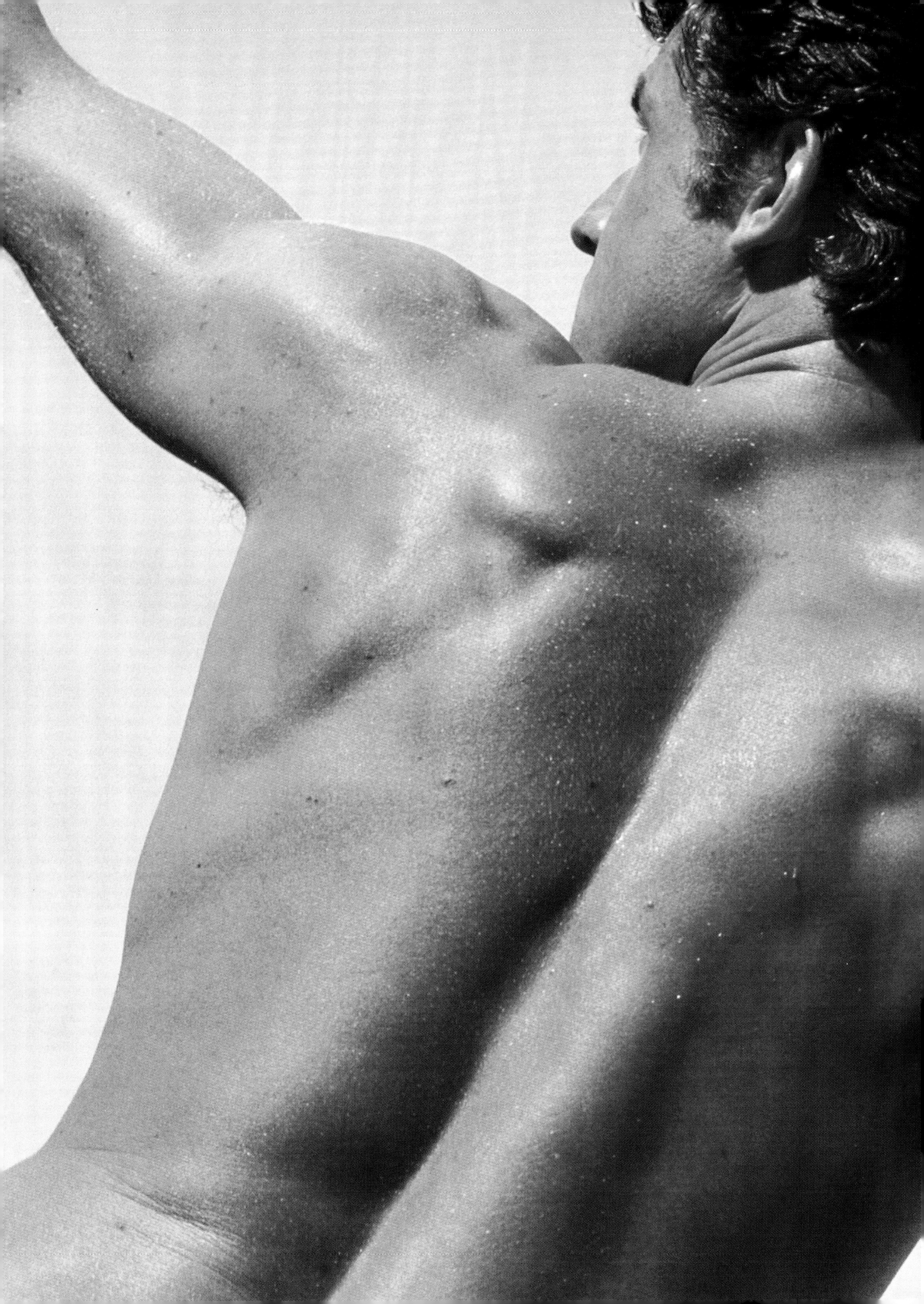

Contents

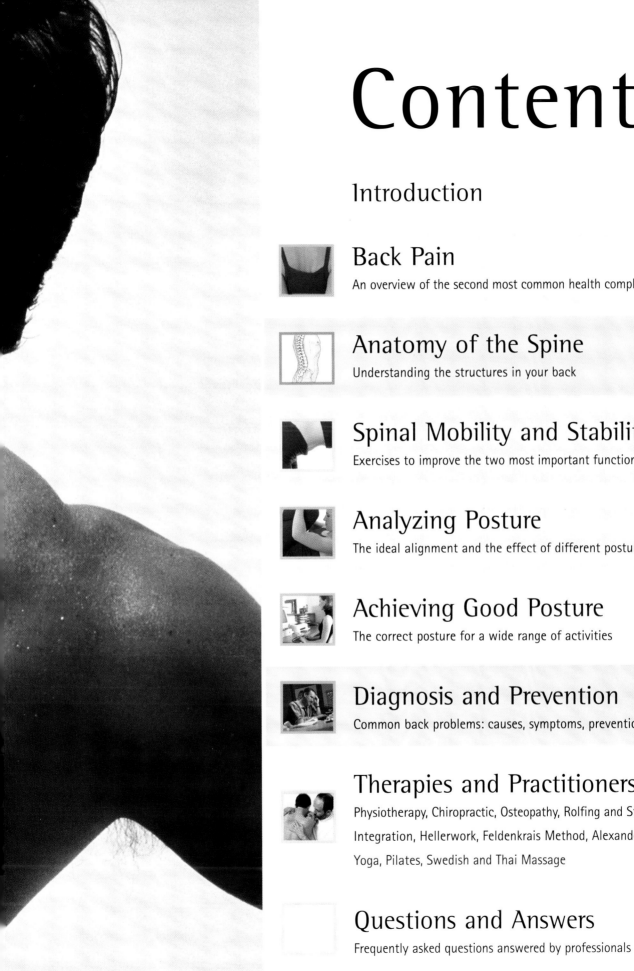

Introduction

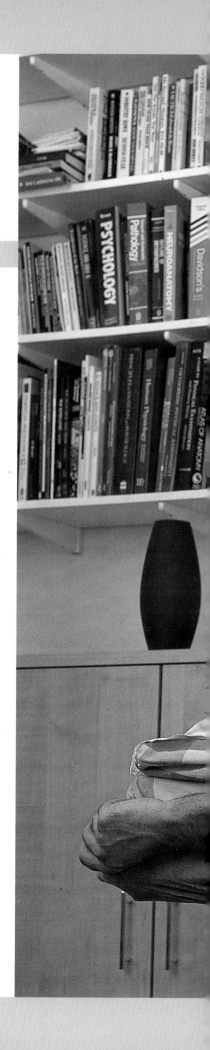

The Good Back Book offers you guidelines to protect your back and to understand conditions under which you will be more prone to injury. It is difficult to lay down a set of circumstances and activities that will improve or prevent back problems, because every back and every back problem is different. Therefore you should understand that these are only recommendations and not hard and fast rules that guarantee 100 percent success. If you already have a back problem it is best to have it evaluated by a professional who can advise you personally on your particular problem.

In this book we present a basic anatomy of the back so that you can become familiar with the structures that can lead to back pain. We discuss the importance of posture and how avoiding or correcting certain movements can prevent back problems. We also present factors that have been shown to be associated with back problems and we offer a number of exercises that may help prevent back strain and lower back pain.

We have taken a conservative approach to dealing with back problems, and adhere to proven medical facts that have been verified through proper research. Because manual therapists such as physiotherapists, chiropractors and osteopaths often have contradicting opinions on prevention, we have also adhered to advice accepted by the majority of professionals.

As with all health problems, it is important that you seek professional medical advice before commencing any exercise or therapy program.

We hope you will enjoy learning more about your back and how to keep it healthy!

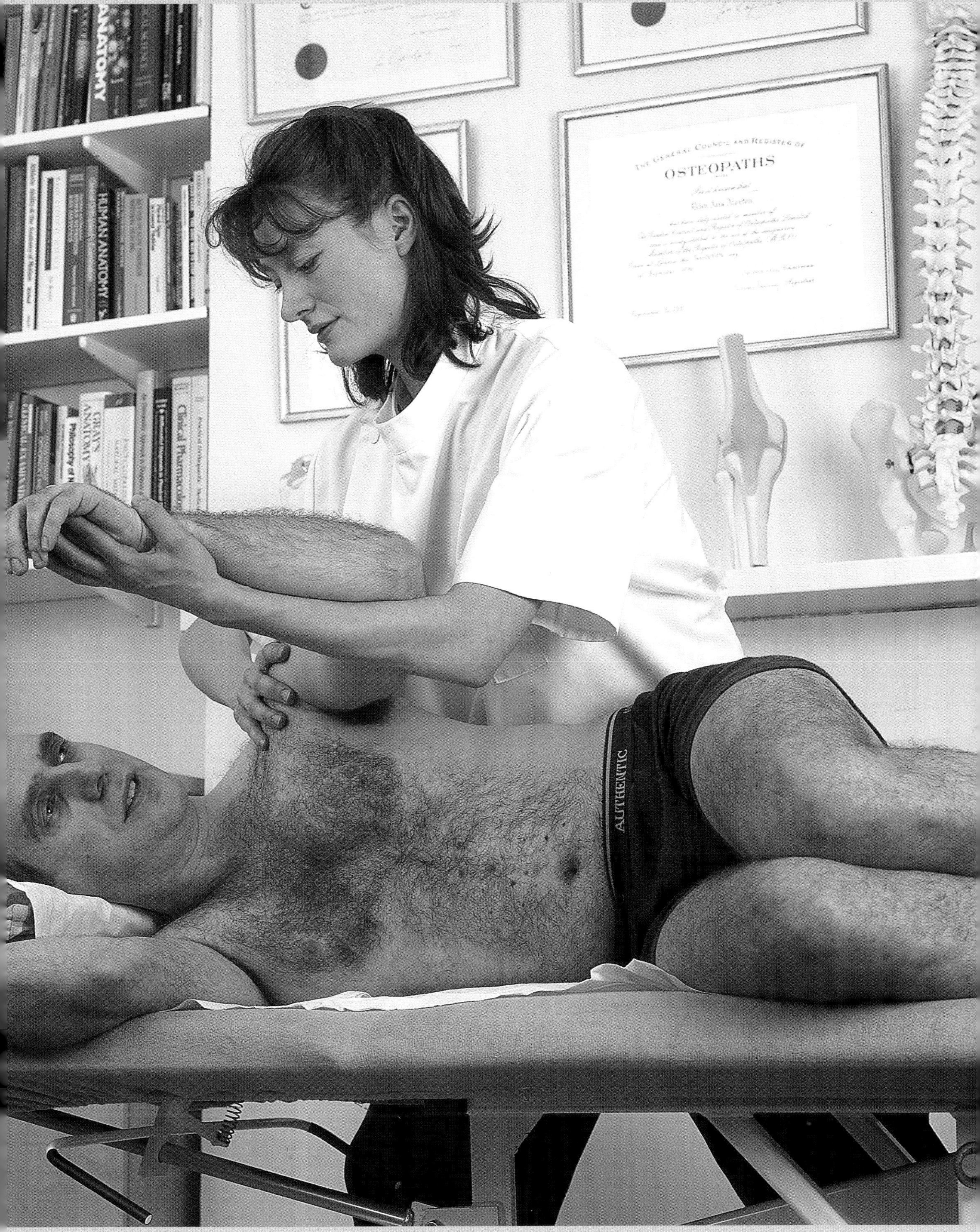
ANATOMY
HUMAN ANATOMY
GRAY'S ANATOMY
THE GENERAL COUNCIL AND REGISTER OF
OSTEOPATHS
AUTHENTIC

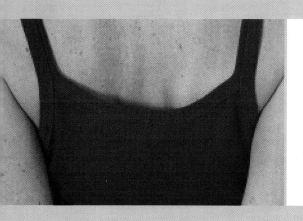

Back Pain
A UNIVERSAL CONCERN

Each year more than 16 million Americans consult their doctors for relief from back pain. While it has no regard for age, race, gender, status or level of education, back pain is related to your genetic inheritance as well as the use and abuse of your back. The type of work and endurance you expect of your back is often unfair, especially when you look at the training you give it to be able to cope with these demands.

You are probably unaware of how your back is affected by day-to-day activities, or how your spine may react to certain movements. Your back has more range of movement than any other part of your body – it can bend forwards, backwards and rotate sideways – and as a result has more potential for injury. The lower back is under the most strain as it must support not only the weight associated with activity, but also the weight of the thorax and ultimately the neck and head, too. The load on your lower back varies substantially according to how you use it. In fact, it is likely that because you are unaware of how to support your spine, you use your back more than you need to. Unfortunately, what you do with your back daily directly impacts on how long it will stay healthy – therefore the more you abuse your spine, e.g. sitting and standing incorrectly or picking things up incorrectly, the more likely you are to injure your back.

Are you the only one with back problems? Definitely not. Surveys have shown that millions of people report back and spine-related problems each year. The following examples will you give you some idea of just how widespread back complaints can be:

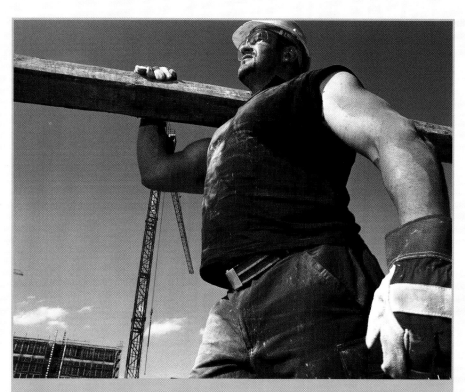

Forced to handle heavy loads on a daily basis, construction workers and manual laborers are a high risk category for back injuries.

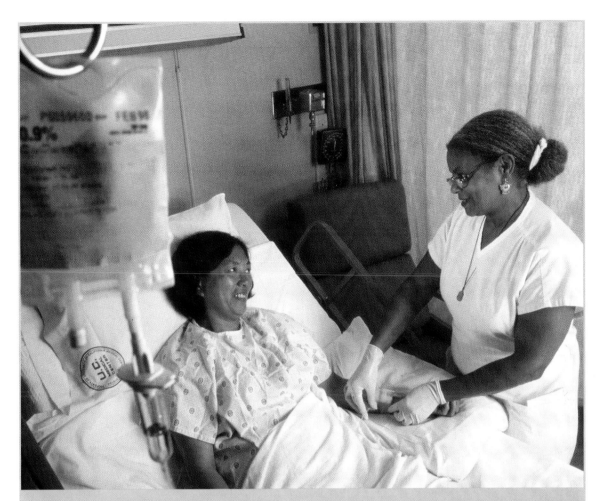

Medical practitioners working long hours, often with no opportunity for rest, may unwittingly put enormous strain on the structures in their back.

- More than 30 percent of all workers compensation costs are related to back injury, making back pain the leading cause of all claims.
- Back pain affects 80 percent of adults and costs the economy more than $20 billion annually (with some estimates exceeding $50 billion) in medical care, workers compensation and time lost from work.
- About two percent of the U.S. population is disabled by back pain.
- People working in heavy industries are subject to back pain, particularly when their job entails any bending and turning motions. For example, bricklayers experience a wide incidence of back problems because of

80 percent of people experience lower back pain at some point in their lives.

their specific back movements (forward bending at the same time as turning, or rotation) and because of their sustained forward bending when mixing cement.

- Nurses have a high incidence of back problems – about four times the national average – because of the physical activity involved in handling patients and the long hours spent on their feet.
- Construction workers, truck drivers, garbage collectors and various types of healthcare workers have some of the highest risk of back injury.
- For sedentary workers, slouching behind a computer or bending over a microscope leads to sustained bad posture, which puts an unnecessary amount of strain on the lower back, inevitably leading to back pain.

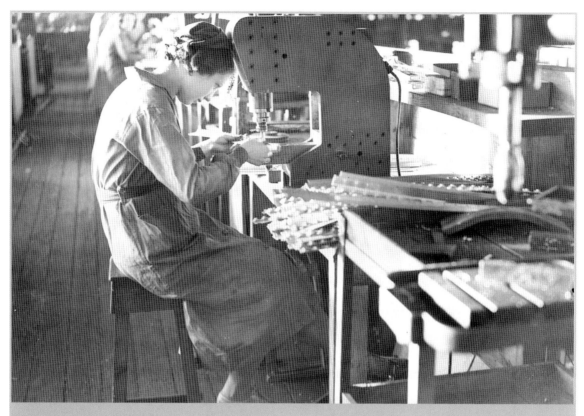

This circa 1920 photograph shows how back problems are not a new complaint, though a worker in a similar situation today would likely have a chair that supports the lower back.

- Factory workers who spend hours working at surfaces that are at an inconvenient height or distance also frequently succumb to back pain. Their daily routine involves leaning over and stretching to reach equipment or merchandise. Sustained stretching puts additional load on the back while it is already strained or incorrectly aligned, making it more prone to injury.

About 80 percent of people will experience lower back problems at some time in their lives. More than 120 million work days are lost annually to backache, and it is the leading cause of workers compensation costs. The hours lost due to sick leave represent substantial financial losses, and this has become a huge problem for industries.

Of all the people experiencing lower back pain for the first time, 60 percent of them will experience their second episode of back pain within a year. Thus, one of the strongest predictors for a new episode of lower back pain is a previous episode. Quite simply, the secret to a healthy back is to aim for prevention rather than cure.

Educating yourself about your back will make you more aware of how it functions optimally and under which circumstances it will not last. Knowing more about your back and back problems may reduce the use of medical services and will certainly decrease your apprehension and speed up recovery. Training your back with specific exercises and changing the way you do things will help to prevent lower back problems and save you time, money and a lot of discomfort.

There are a number of factors that increase the risk of developing lower back problems. Some of the most common ones are listed below.

LIFESTYLE

A balanced lifestyle includes moderate exercise and fitness, mobility and cardiovascular fitness. These elements have a positive effect on the whole body. A balanced lifestyle makes your heart stronger, decreases cholesterol, reduces the risk of cardiovascular problems, increases the muscle support to the spine and, last but not least, it reduces the risk of developing lower back pain. Increasingly, lower back pain seems to develop because

Other factors that have been known to contribute to back pain include:

- Weak abdominal muscles
- General muscular tension
- Depression
- Emotional distress
- Excess weight
- Absence of regular exercise
- Job dissatisfaction
- Job ergonomics

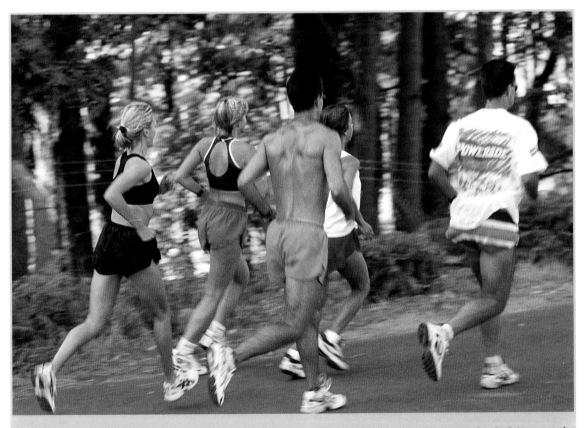

A balanced lifestyle should include a moderate amount of exercise — too much, and the body's natural defenses are compromised.

of the sedentary lifestyles we lead, due to the convenience of modern living and because both the young and old have become less active.

A balanced lifestyle also includes a balanced dietary pattern. An unhealthy diet can lead to weight problems that contribute to extra stress on the spine. As your muscles weaken, you develop bad posture, putting further strain on your back. Numerous studies also indicate that smoking increases the risk of developing lower back pain because it speeds up the degenerative process. This will most probably include disc problems.

STRESS

There are two different types of stress that can affect your back: emotional (or psychological) stress and mechanical stress. An emotionally stressed person undergoes certain physical changes. Posture is affected, putting more pressure on the ligaments, joints and muscles, making them more susceptible to mechanical strain. Studies have shown that psychological stress can increase compression and lateral shear in a spinal joint, which in turn increases the risk of lower back pain. In cases of existing lower back pain, occupational stress aggravates it further.

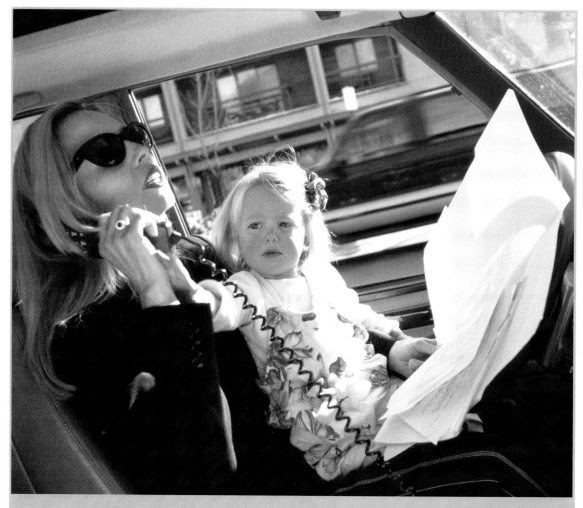

The demands of being a "perfect mother" — working mothers are exposed to both emotional and mechanical stress.

People who are overweight or use their back incorrectly can also experience mechanical stress on their spine. Different positions create a variety of forces on the spine, but remaining in one position increases the stress on the lower back. This leads to irritation, and over a long period of time, to degenerative changes in the structure of the spine.

GRAVITY

Through gravity you experience compression of your joints. However, not all compression is harmful. Active compression when the spinal column is in a good posture is necessary to keep your bone density high, and your bones in a healthy condition, helping to prevent osteoporosis and reduce the risk of developing spinal fractures. Intermittent ("pump action") compression is also essential, as it

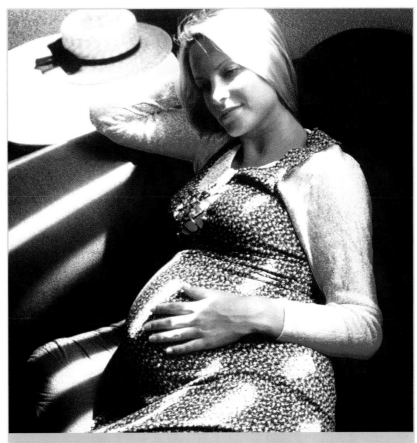

Additional physical weight affects pregnant or overweight individuals by lengthening the supporting abdominal muscles and compromising the stability of the spine.

maintains the movement of fluid in the spinal joint, bringing in nutrients, removing waste products and keeping the joint lubricated for ease of movement. Constant sustained compression in a bad posture (e.g. sitting slumped over, walking in a forward bending position), on the other hand, is not good for the joints. It presses out the fluids in the intervertebral discs and cartilage of the joint, leaving them relatively dehydrated and more vulnerable to tears.

PREGNANCY AND WEIGHT PROBLEMS

Pregnancy and gaining weight go hand in hand. Pregnant women pick up a considerable amount of weight in a relatively short period of time, and the body is forced to adjust quickly. Increase in weight and size mostly to the

front of the body, hollows the lower spine and causes the joints to close and compress onto each other. Because of the extra load and girth, the abdominal muscles supporting the lower back become weak, resulting in reduced support to the spine. The joints take more strain as they deal with an ever-increasing load. Overweight people undergo similar physical changes and suffer the same consequences.

Another factor that plays a role during pregnancy is the increased production of hormones, which have a relaxing (or lengthening) effect on the ligaments in preparation for childbirth. This lengthening occurs in all the ligaments, and as a result those ligaments that play a role in stabilizing the spine may become compromised.

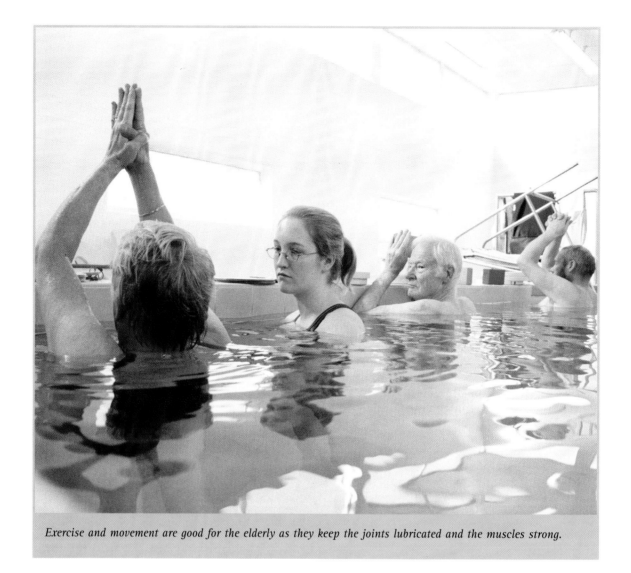

Exercise and movement are good for the elderly as they keep the joints lubricated and the muscles strong.

AGE

With age, changes occur in the vertebral column — the joint cartilage thins and becomes more brittle, joints may become increasingly stiff and there is a decreased range of movement. Age-related changes do not necessarily mean that you will experience pain or discomfort; they do, however, make you more vulnerable to injury. Sustained incorrect use of your back may also lead to complications as you get older, and will certainly speed up the degenerative changes. The chances of experiencing lower back problems are greatly increased between the ages of 55 and 64. The length of the vertebral column decreases with age because of the gradual wear of the vertebral end plates, which is associated with the reduction of bone density (osteoporosis). This usually appears earlier in women than in men, and is often associated with middle age and menopausal changes. However, bone loss as a result of aging is not inevitable. Some of it may be difficult to avoid, but with regular exercise and an adequate calcium intake you can reduce or prevent some of the bone loss associated with aging.

WHAT SHOULD YOU DO IF YOU'VE JUST INJURED YOUR BACK?

Back injuries often occur due to repetitive movements or as a consequence of maintaining a fixed position. They are also more likely to occur when an action is done quickly, without thinking. The best thing to do immediately after sustaining a back injury is to stop the activity that you are engaged in. Try to bend your back in the opposite position to the one you've been working in, but stop immediately if it hurts. Try sitting if it gives you relief. Alternatively, find a comfortable position and maintain a gentle and slow movement cycle.

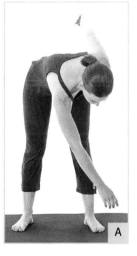

Disc injuries often happen when bending forward and simultaneously twisting to the side A . If you can manage it, you may want to kneel on your hands and knees and move your back B . Hollowing and rounding movements can often provide relief from back pain.

Another option would be to lie down after the injury for approximately 30 minutes. A good position to relieve back strain involves lying on your back with your knees bent at 90 degrees, your legs resting on a few pillows (see page 81, figure B). If the pain subsides and you can stand up without discomfort, you should be able to go back to work, but avoid activities that cause pain. If you still experience discomfort it would be advisable to rest your back for the remainder of the day and stay away from the activity that caused your injury. You should see a doctor, if possible. If, after the injury, you can barely move and the pain is very acute, it is advisable to see a doctor as soon as possible.

If you wake up in the morning with acute pain and are unsure of the cause, it could be as a result of an injury sustained the previous day — the swelling would have appeared during the night, causing you to feel pain. A doctor can prescribe medication for the inflammation and will probably refer you to a manual therapist for treatment (i.e., physiotherapist, chiropractor, etc.).

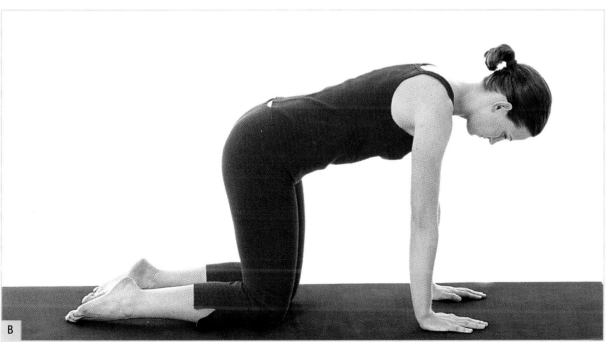

WHEN SHOULD YOU CONSULT A DOCTOR?

- When you have back pain for longer than a day without any sign of improvement.
- When you have chronic (long-lasting) back pain.
- When you have minor back pain that lasts for longer than 4–5 days.
- When you have pain in your back and pain down the leg (radiating pain).
- When you have pain down the leg or loss of sensation (feeling) in your leg or foot that you have never experienced previously.
- When you experience difficulty in walking and you relate it to your back, especially when a leg or foot feels weak.
- When you experience "pins and needles" in your leg.
- When you experience prolonged or repeated pins and needles in both legs at the same time, and it lasts longer than a few minutes.
- When you start developing a problem with your bladder or bowel, or even a loss of feeling between your legs that you've never experienced before.

WHEN SHOULD YOU SEE A PHYSIOTHERAPIST, A CHIROPRACTOR OR AN OSTEOPATH?

The one thing these professions have in common is that they are qualified to evaluate a musculoskeletal problem; and they often have a better understanding of the type of injury than a general practitioner would. This does not mean that the doctor plays any less of a role; he or she will make sure the problem is of a mechanical nature and eliminate other potential causes of the pain. If your doctor is sure the problem is mechanical, he or she will refer you to a manual therapist.

Physiotherapists and osteopaths use joint mobilizing techniques and manipulation as well as massage and various other methods of soft tissue (i.e. muscles and ligaments) treatment. They work on the structures actually causing discomfort and the underlying structures that are often the primary cause of the problem. They also deal with preventive treatment to avoid the re-occurrence of the problem. Osteopaths and chiropractors use quick manipulation to correct the alignment of the spine, bringing balance back into the spinal structures and the structures around them.

All these professionals are qualified to evaluate your problem and treat you accordingly, though the medical community cannot always agree on their efficacy. You will need to find what works best for you. (*See* Chapter 7 – Therapies and Practitioners for more information.)

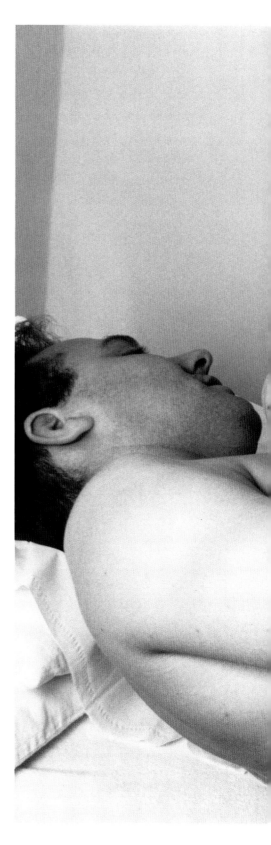

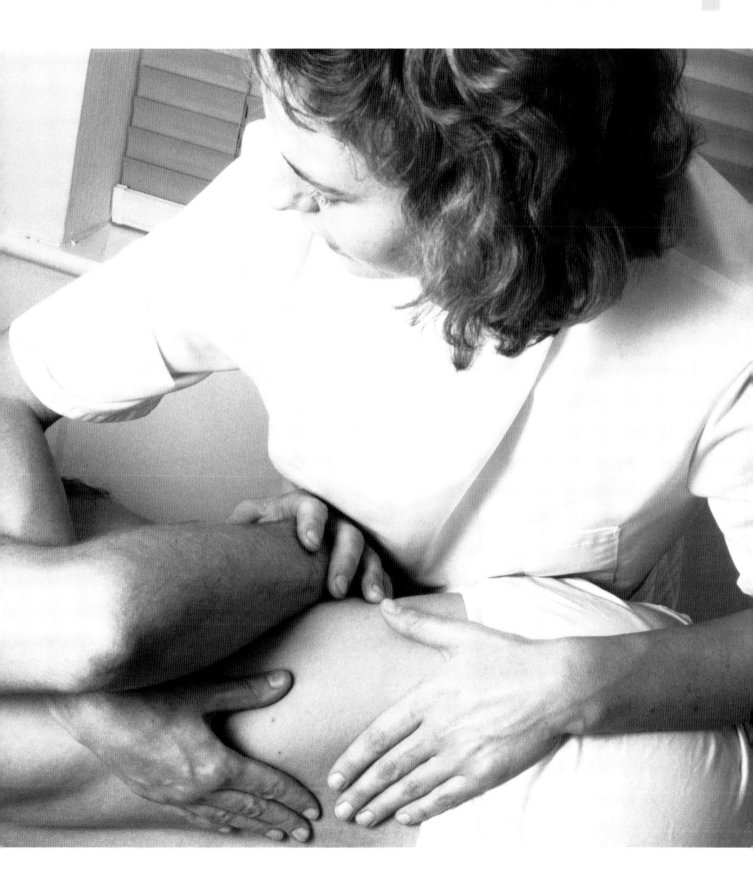

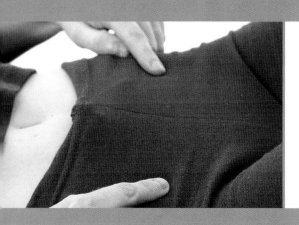

Anatomy
of the Spine

The vertebral column is a structure unlike any other in the body. It has two main functions: firstly to move, and to have enough mobility to perform certain activities, and secondly, to provide a stable base that supports the upper and lower limbs allowing them to function effectively. For a healthy body to work as a whole, the vertebral column needs to be able to perform both these functions properly. If it lacks either of these qualities it is more prone to injury. In order to prevent injury you need to understand the structures in your back and how they function. This next section will give you an idea of what these structures are, what they look like and how they work.

THE VERTEBRAL COLUMN

The vertebral column, the most important component in the back, goes through three developmental stages: the blastemal, cartilaginous and osseous stages. The blastemal stage develops in utero at three weeks; at this stage the column is actually just a cord and extremely soft. The cartilaginous stage begins in utero at two months, and at this point the

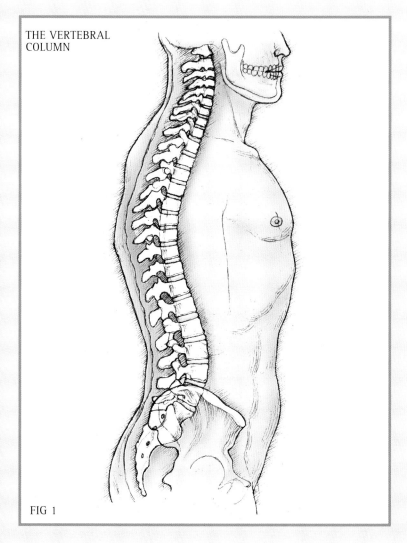

THE VERTEBRAL
COLUMN

FIG 1

vertebral bodies start to form. Finally, during the osseous stage, blood vessels grow into the cartilaginous vertebrae as centers of hard bone appear. The entire vertebra ossifies (becomes bone) except for the growth,

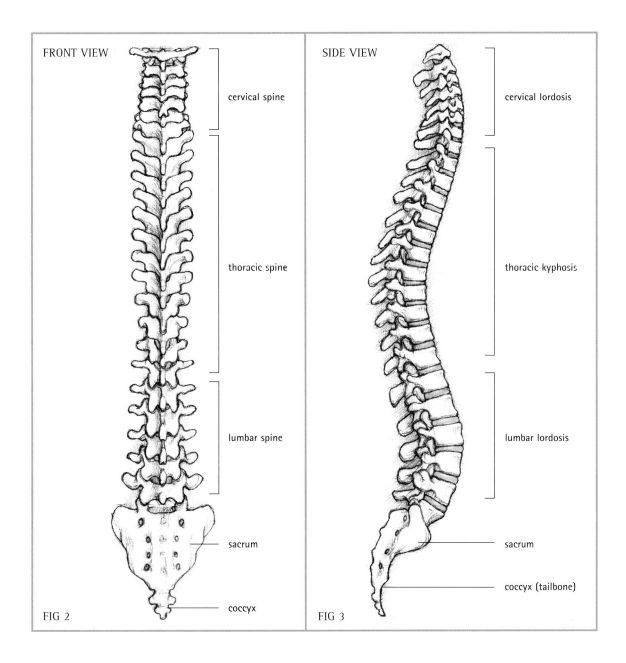

FRONT VIEW

cervical spine

thoracic spine

lumbar spine

sacrum

coccyx

FIG 2

SIDE VIEW

cervical lordosis

thoracic kyphosis

lumbar lordosis

sacrum

coccyx (tailbone)

FIG 3

or end plates, which lie on either extreme — these remain cartilaginous virtually throughout life.

The vertebral column is made up of 33 vertebrae stacked one on top of another (see fig 1). Twenty-four are individual vertebrae; five of the remaining nine are fused to form the sacrum; and the last four form the coccygeal vertebrae commonly referred to as the coccyx or tailbone. The vertebrae fit into one another like a puzzle, with an intervertebral disc between each piece, except for the top two which have a specialized structure that serves to support the skull. The entire column is divided into three main sections, the neck (cervical), the trunk (thoracic) and the lower back (lumbar) area. There are seven neck vertebrae, 12 trunk vertebrae and five lower back vertebrae. Below the lower back vertebrae lies the sacral bone, a solid triangular piece of bone at the back of the pelvis, and below that the coccyx (see fig 2).

The vertebral column has several curves along its length. In the neck and lower back there is a slight hollowing, known as cervical and lumbar lordosis, respectively, and in the trunk there is a rounding, or thoracic kyphosis (see fig 3). Many people think that a spine must be ramrod straight, but this is an incorrect assumption. Lordosis and kyphosis are normal components of a healthy spine; however, excessive hollowing or rounding can lead to complications.

THE LUMBAR VERTEBRAE

Five vertebrae make up the lower back section of the spine, known as L1-L5 (see fig 4). The vertebrae here are considerably larger than in the neck and trunk. This is because the lower back carries a bigger load than the neck and is shaped to support the weight of the upper body and its movement.

Front and back components make up each lumbar vertebra. The front component, or the vertebral body, is a flat, oval-shaped structure, shaped in this way so that it can stack easily and bear weight. The back component is a triangular-shaped structure with a central canal that protects the spinal cord. Bony wings at either side are known as the transverse processes and a central protrusion, called the spinous process, extends backwards forming the bumps that you can see running down your back (see fig 5.1). Viewed from the side, the back component has additional bony protrusions, known as the facets. These form synovial joints similar to the knuckle or knee joints and serve to link the spinal vertebrae together so that they stay in place.

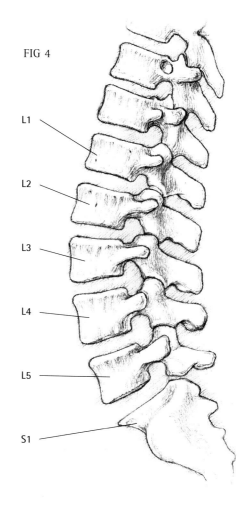

FIG 4

L1

L2

L3

L4

L5

S1

LUMBAR VERTEBRA

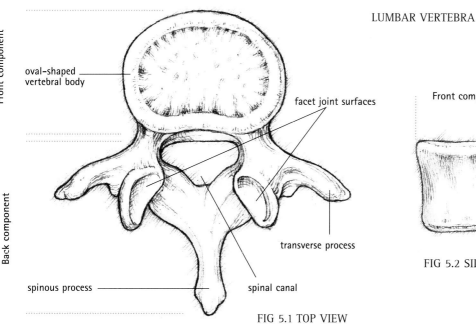

Front component

Back component

oval–shaped vertebral body

facet joint surfaces

transverse process

spinous process

spinal canal

FIG 5.1 TOP VIEW

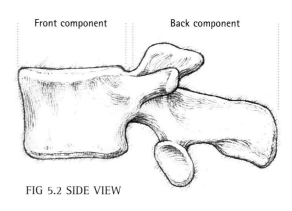

Front component

Back component

FIG 5.2 SIDE VIEW

THE INTERVERTEBRAL DISCS

The vertebrae are prevented from grinding against one another by oval-shaped intervertebral discs. These are essentially pressure pillows that lie on the vertebral body and help to absorb weight and pressure.

THE INTERVERTEBRAL DISCS

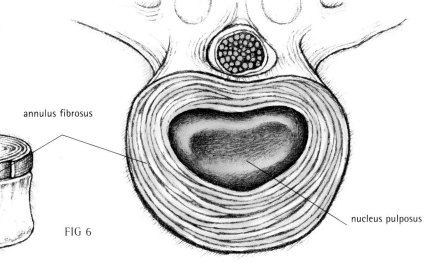

annulus fibrosus

nucleus pulposus

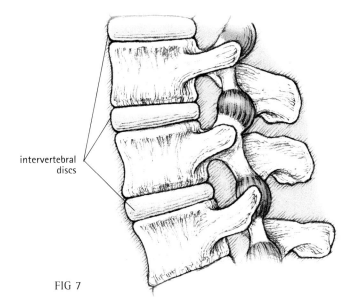

FIG 6

Each intervertebral disc consists of two different types of structures. If you were to cut a transverse slice through a disc and look at it from the top, you would see an outer and an inner structure (see fig 6). The outer part, called the annulus fibrosus, is a fibrous cartilage layer, arranged in onion-like layers around the inner part. The inner part, or nucleus pulposus, is a gel-like structure that consists of 88 percent water, which gives it a pliable nature. The gel lies slightly to the back of the disc, and as a result the annulus fibrosus is thickest and strongest in the front. The weakest part of the annulus is at the back, which is where it is most likely to tear.

The function of the intervertebral discs is to absorb and distribute shock and the weight of the upper body, as well as any extra load held or carried. When the lower back moves the gel changes shape and, depending on the movement, there is extra stretch on specific areas of the annulus.

Internal disc pressure, or the load that the disc has to absorb, varies according to its position in the column and the position of your back. Different postures place different types of strain on the discs. The study in the

intervertebral discs

FIG 7

diagram on the next page (see fig 9) illustrates the pressure on an intervertebral disc in the lower back resulting from different postures. The diagram shows that the pressure is less in the lying position than in the standing position. It shows that it is even less when standing than sitting. Any forward bending increases the pressure in the disc quite dramatically.

During a normal day's activity, the body's weight puts pressure on the discs causing some of the water content in the nucleus to dissipate and become absorbed by the structures around it (see fig 8); as a result the intervertebral discs become thinner in the daytime. When you lie down and remove the compression load off the discs, the water content is restored. If your disc is damaged, the inflammation can increase the internal pressure, limiting movement. This is why you sometimes feel stiff in the morning; it is also why you are most prone to injury when you first get up.

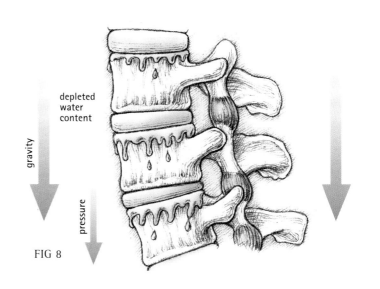

depleted water content

gravity

pressure

FIG 8

FIG 9 PRESSURE ON THE INVERTEBRAL DISC IN A VARIETY OF DIFFERENT POSITIONS
Source: *Neck and Back Pain*, Nachemson and Jonsson.
Lippincott, Williams and Wilkin (2000)

It is interesting to note that sitting puts more strain on the lower back than standing. The pressure on the intervertebral disc is futher increased in the forward bending position and is even higher when lifting or simultaneously lifting and twisting. These activities are high-risk categories when it comes to disc damage and degeneration.

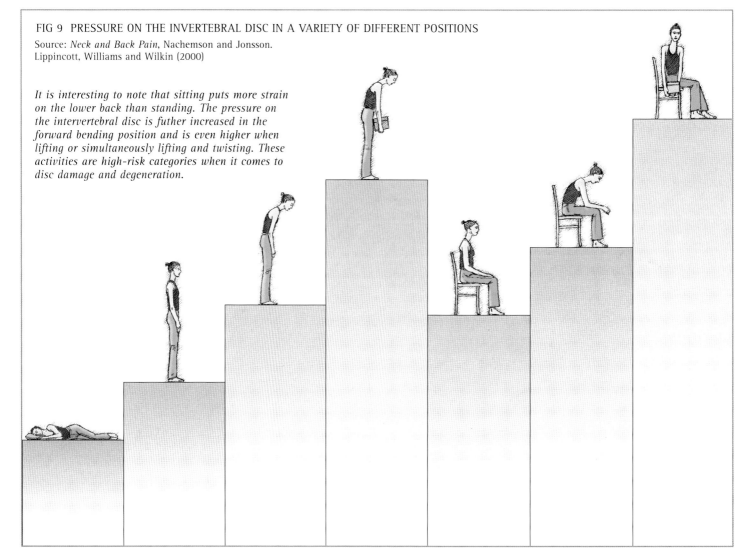

The water content of the nucleus becomes depleted with age, making it less pliable and more resistant to movement. Because of the decreased disc motility, other structures — ligaments, muscles and joints — are forced to compensate and can become more stressed. This stress can cause injury to the structures that are compensating.

THE FACET JOINTS

The back component of each vertebra has two pairs of bony protrusions known as facet joints, one pair facing upward, the other downward, on each side of the vertebra (see fig 10.1 and 10.2). Facet joints are plate-like structures that link the vertebrae together. Each joint consists of two bony processes lined with cartilage, enabling the joints to move or glide (articulate) smoothly against each other. A capsule containing synovial fluid encloses the joint surfaces, providing lubrication as well as nutrition to the joint cartilage (see fig 10.3).

The angle of the facet joints varies along the vertebral column, contributing to its ability to regulate or control movement. This is particularly important when it comes to forward and backward movement. With forward bending, the top facets glide forward and tip upward, separating from the lower facets and forming a gap between the joint. The capsule stretches to accommodate this action, while at the same time preventing an excessive range of movement. If the movement is repeatedly done incorrectly, or to an extreme, the capsule can become overstretched and lose its ability to contain movement.

Facet joints contribute toward regulating movement.

With backward bending, the facets from the superior bone glide down onto the facets of the inferior bone. The tension in the periarticular structures — the capsule and the ligaments — increases progressively as a result of the backward movement; this, together with the increased tension in the intervertebral disc, has the effect of restricting an excess range of backward bending. (See next page for more on range of movement.)

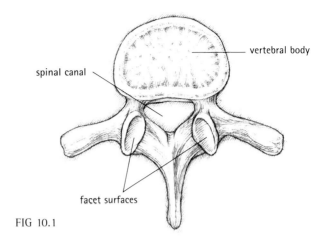

FIG 10.1

spinal canal
vertebral body
facet surfaces

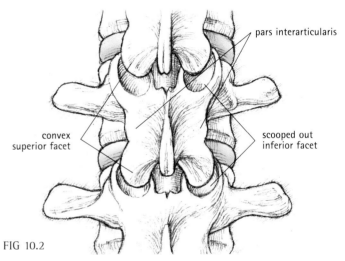

FIG 10.2

pars interarticularis
convex superior facet
scooped out inferior facet

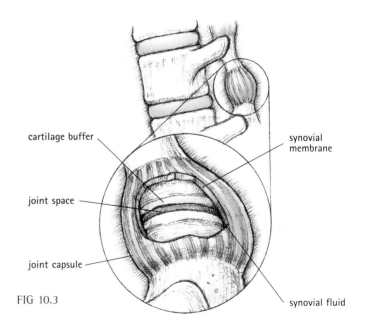

FIG 10.3

cartilage buffer
joint space
joint capsule
synovial membrane
synovial fluid

Range of movement

The back has a large range of movement, more so than any other structure in the body; it can move forward, backwards, sideways and rotate, and as such is at greater risk to injury. Normal specific movements are vital to the health of the structures in the back, and the maintenance of mobility. If the back is maintained in one position for long periods of time, or excessively moved in any direction, it becomes damaging to the structures.

Flexion (bending forward)

When bending forward, the lower back flattens out losing its normal curve. The gel of the intervertebral disc is driven back increasing the pressure on the rear of the disc, the weakest part of the annulus fibrosus. The top facet moves upwards, away from the bottom facet (see fig 11), stretching the capsular ligaments. Repetitive forward bending is a common cause of disc problems.

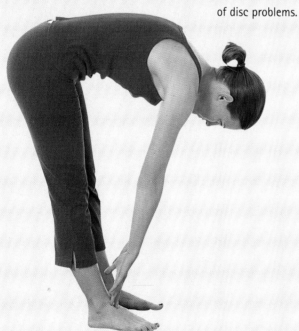

Side flexion (bending sideways)

The top facet slides and compresses over the bottom facet on the side towards which the movement is taking place. On the opposite side, the facet opens up and the ligaments and muscles stretch. There is an increase of pressure on the intervertebral disc on the side towards which the movement occurs (see fig 12). Excessive sideways movement can overstretch structures such as the ligaments and the muscles on the opposite side of the movement. The facet joint on the same side of the movement may also be compressed and suffer injury.

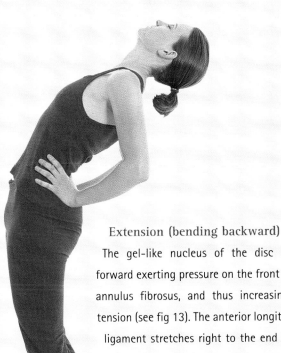

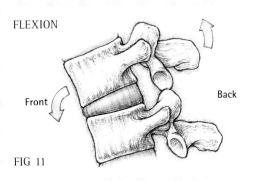

FLEXION

Front

Back

FIG 11

Extension (bending backward)

The gel-like nucleus of the disc moves forward exerting pressure on the front of the annulus fibrosus, and thus increasing the tension (see fig 13). The anterior longitudinal ligament stretches right to the end of the movement and the facet joints compress onto one another. Excessive backwards movement usually injures the facet joints due to too much compression.

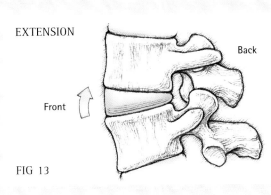

SIDE FLEXION

FIG 12

Rotation (twisting your back)

The facet joints, which compress on the side to which the rotation is taking place and open on the side from which the movement stems, restrict movement at the end of a rotation (see fig 14). The ligaments around the outer layer of the intervertebral disc also contribute to stopping further movement. If a rotation movement goes too far it often causes an injury to the annulus fibrosus.

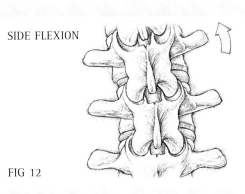

EXTENSION

Back

Front

FIG 13

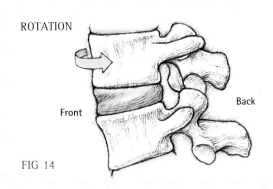

ROTATION

Front

Back

FIG 14

LIGAMENTS

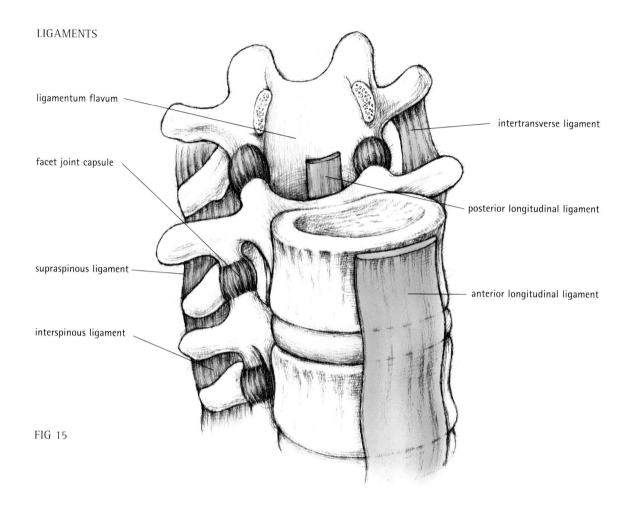

ligamentum flavum

intertransverse ligament

facet joint capsule

posterior longitudinal ligament

supraspinous ligament

anterior longitudinal ligament

interspinous ligament

FIG 15

LIGAMENTS

Ligaments are fibrous bands or sheets of connective tissue linking two or more bones, cartilages or structures together. While ligaments are not able to control movement, they do play an important part in preventing excessive range of movement in flexion, extension and rotation.

You have six main ligaments in your back, all of which are associated with the intervertebral disc and the facet joint movements (see fig 15). These structures are usually divided into two groups, the ligaments between vertebrae (interspinous, intertransverse and ligamentum flavum) and ligaments that span a group of vertebrae (supraspinous, anterior and posterior longitudinal). The ligamentum flavum, which lies inside the spinal canal, consists of a great number of elastic fibers making it extremely flexible. This and the other ligaments play an important role in the stability of the vertebral column both in motion and at rest. Total support of the vertebral column, however, requires muscular assistance.

MUSCLES

The primary function of the large lateral muscles in the back (erector spinae group) is to move the spine. The smaller, deeper muscles closer to the vertebral column, on the other hand, play an important role in stabilizing the vertebral column. It is vitally important to maintain the stabilizing action of the muscles for a healthy back. People with lower back problems tend to use their stabilizing muscles incorrectly or not at all.

The antero-lateral group of abdominal muscles (including the external and internal obliques, the rectus abdominus and the transverse abdominus) also play an important part in stabilizing the spine. Of these, the deep abdominal muscle, the transverse abdominus, is perhaps the most important stabilizer. The transverse abdominus lies below your navel and extends across your abdomen from side to side (see fig 16.1). The thoraco-lumbar fascia is an important link between the transverse abdominus and the spine. It is a tight, flat band spanning the lower back, which attaches to the spinous process of each vertebra (see fig 16.2). The transverse abdominal muscles have an attachment to the thoraco-lumbar fascia. When you contract the transverse abdominal muscle, it tightens the tho-

The big moving muscles of the spine can be divided into groups according to the actions they perform:

- Muscles that lie at the back of the spine usually bend the back backwards.
- Abdominal muscles and hip flexors bend the back forwards.
- Muscles on the sides of the spine will bend the back sideways or rotate the spine.

raco-lumbar fascia and creates a corset-like effect. By helping the thoraco-lumbar fascia maintain the normal curve in the lower back, the transverse abdominus has a stabilizing effect on the lower back.

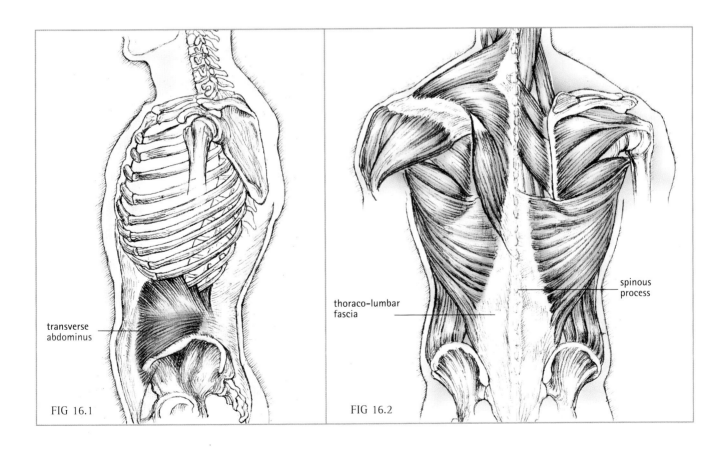

transverse abdominus

FIG 16.1

thoraco-lumbar fascia

spinous process

FIG 16.2

NEURAL STRUCTURES: THE SPINAL CORD AND SPINAL NERVES

Nerves carry messages from the brain, through the spinal cord, to specific structures in the body. The nerves form nerve endings in a structure, which emit and receive impulses (messages) to and from the brain. Structures that have nerve endings can feel pain, while those without nerve endings are immune to pain.

The spinal cord is protected by the vertebral bones and an encapsulating sheath called the dura mater. Spinal nerves (see fig 17), also protected by a sheath, leave the spinal cord through the intervertebral foramen, small gaps in-between the vertebrae. Part of the spinal nerve returns to the vertebrae and all the structures around the vertebrae, including the facet joints. The rest forms part of two nerve plexuses, the lumbar plexus and the sacral plexus. The femoral nerve (see fig 18), which arises from the lumbar plexus, extends down the thigh, supplying the front of the leg while the sciatic nerve (see fig 19), which stems from the sacral plexus, runs down the back of the leg all the way to the foot.

The spinal nerves are sometimes injured or trapped (impinged) in the intervertebral canal as they leave the vertebra. Other structures, such as muscles and/or ligaments, can put pressure on the sheath anywhere along the pathway of the nerve. Nerve compression causes what is known as a radiating pain; for example, pain that is felt down the length of the leg in the case of the sciatic nerve. Nerve pain can be extreme and may give a feeling of "pins and needles" in the foot. It can also weaken muscles in the legs and make your skin feel different to that of the other foot. Should femoral and/or sciatic nerves become injured they can, in most cases, heal if the problem is managed correctly. However, an important preventive measure is to keep the protective sheaths mobile and healthy. (See pp44–45 for specific neural mobility exercises.)

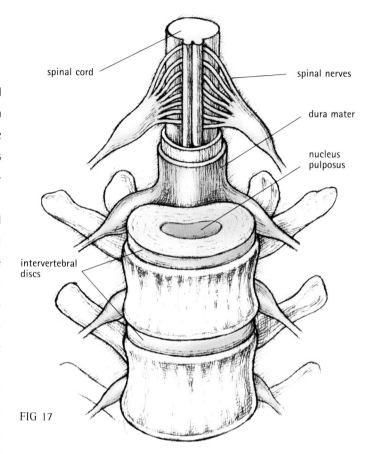

spinal cord

spinal nerves

dura mater

nucleus pulposus

intervertebral discs

FIG 17

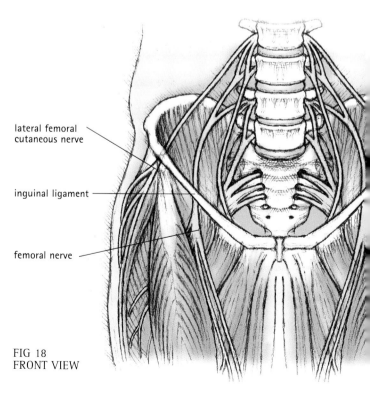

lateral femoral cutaneous nerve

inguinal ligament

femoral nerve

FIG 18
FRONT VIEW

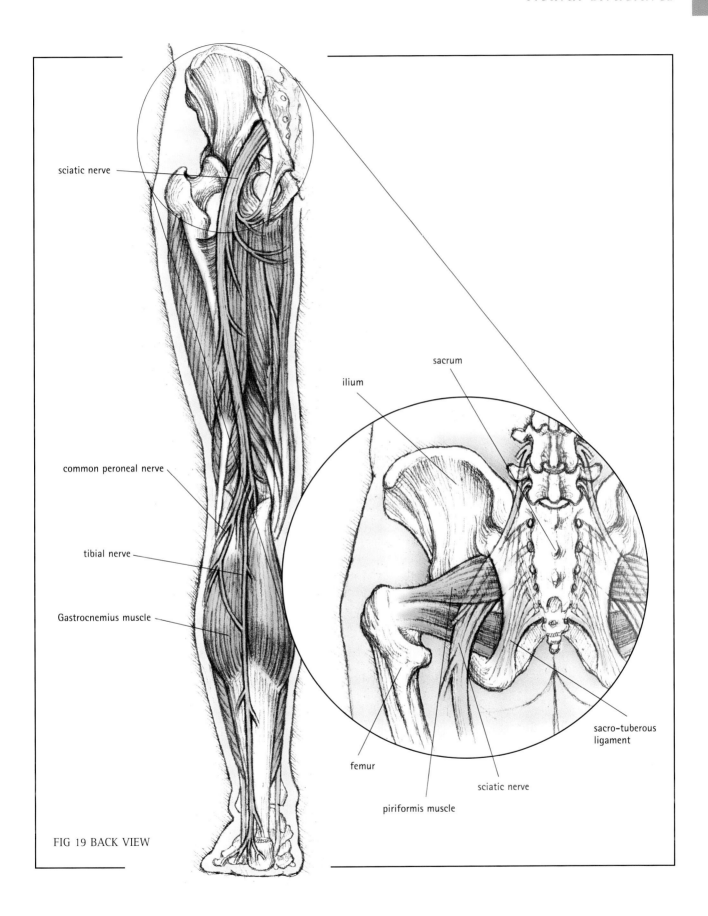

sciatic nerve

common peroneal nerve

tibial nerve

Gastrocnemius muscle

FIG 19 BACK VIEW

ilium

sacrum

femur

piriformis muscle

sciatic nerve

sacro-tuberous
ligament

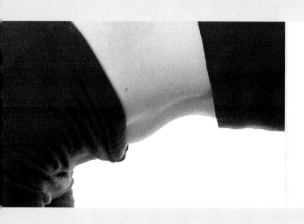

Spinal Mobility and Stability

The balance between the mobility and the stability of the vertebral column is of immense importance to a healthy back. While the column must be mobile, it also requires a good support structure to stabilize it in the correct posture. For this purpose, the column has passive as well as active sytems.

The passive system consists of the vertebrae, ligaments and capsules; the active system consists of the muscles. These two systems affect both the mobility and the stability of the vertebral column.

The vertebral column must allow for mobility and at the same time provide stability.

It is an interesting fact that the joints as well as the discs depend on movement for good nutrition. The fluid of the joints contains nutrition for the cartilage. Movement not only keeps the joint surfaces lubricated, it also increases the exchange of fluids in and out of the joints, allowing them to absorb nutrients and expel waste products. Movement promotes good blood circulation around the joints, which increases the general health of the structures around the joints. Regular but moderate movement is extremely important to keep the vertebral column in a good working condition.

MOBILITY

A mobile vertebral column means a column in which one can move each level to its full potential. This potential is slightly different for each level of the column. The trunk (thoracic) areas, for example, are less mobile than the neck (cervical) and lower back (lumbar). There is a fine balance between being mobile and being too mobile (hypermobile). Certain athletes, such as gymnasts or ballet dancers, often have a problem with hypermobility in certain areas of their vertebral column, usually in their lower back. This excess mobility allows the facet joints to move too far and too often, exposing them to extreme stresses and making them more prone to injury. With this type of problem the active system (stabilizing muscles) may become strained from overuse and fail to support the joints sufficiently.

The opposite can also occur, i.e. there can be too little or limited movement of the vertebral column. Limited movement will make the joints stiff. Joints affected in this manner are called hypomobile joints. As the passive system (vertebrae, capsules and ligments) stiffens up, so do all the structures around it. As a result, both the active and the passive systems are affected. Hypomobile areas usually develop in people who allow their vertebral columns to remain in incorrect postural positions for long periods of time. Every time you carry out an activity where you need to move your vertebral column to its limit, you stand a chance of straining (or overstretching) the passive and/or active structures in the hypomobile area. A stiff passive and active system can increase compression on the joints causing more wear and tear when they move. It can also lead to inflammation and irritation in the joints and soft tissue around the strained area. These symptoms are similar to those brought about by arthritis.

Mobility of the vertebral column is therefore of utmost importance. Too little mobility can be improved by manual therapy but too much mobility needs to be protected with stabilizing muscle activity. The exercises in this chapter address both of these problems.

STABILITY

Using your body incorrectly or doing activities the wrong way will place more stress on certain areas of the vertebral column than others. Failure to use the most important stabilizing muscle, the transverse abdominus, will allow certain areas of your vertebral column to move too much.

To prevent the joints from becoming too mobile the body must use the active system to support the vertebral column. Correctly contracted, the transverse abdominus prevents excessive, unnecessary movement in the vertebral column, especially the lower back, while the arms and legs remain mobile. The effectiveness of your stabilizers can be affected by misuse or injury, and if the vertebral column is not stable while the limbs are moving, the limbs themselves may become less effective.

The passive system (vertebrae, capsules and ligaments) gives the vertebral column some support, but if the active system does not provide the main support and keep the column correctly aligned, then the passive system begins to take strain and the joints, ligaments and capsules can become compromised.

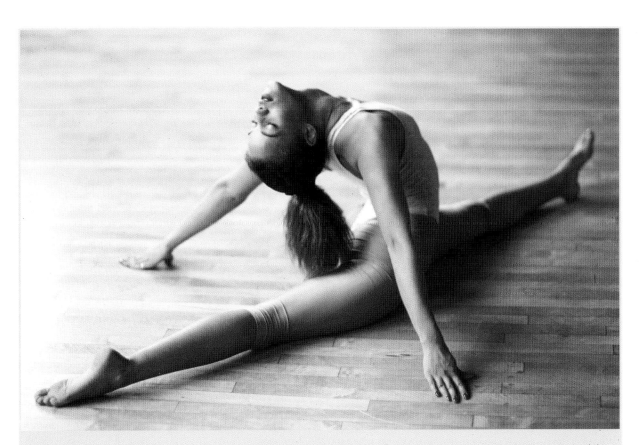

Due to excessive range of movement, gymnasts put extreme strain on their passive support structures, compromising the stability of the spine. Ideally, they should work hard to strengthen the active system, i.e. the transverse abdominus.

MOBILIZING YOUR BACK AND RELATED STRUCTURES

While a good night's sleep will leave you feeling rested, it does mean that the structures in your back have been dormant for six to eight hours and are stiff as a result. It is important that you prepare your back for the day's activities by mobilizing and stretching important muscles and neural structures. For great results do all, not just some, of these quick, easy and effective exercises before you get out of bed.

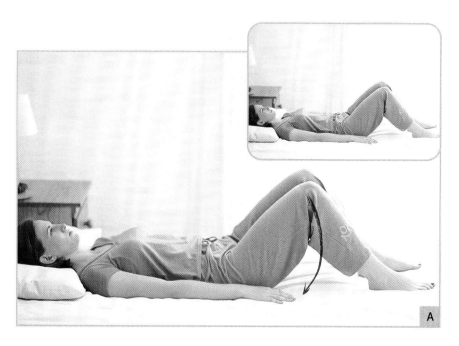

Mobilizing your lower back

Lie on your back with your knees bent and your feet flat on the bed A. Slowly roll your knees from side to side, resting briefly each time your legs reach the midpoint. You should feel some "pull" around the lower back on the opposite side to where your knees roll, but you should not feel any pain on the side toward which the movement takes place. Do five to 10 repetitions of this exercise.

Mobilizing the neural structures and the lower vertebral joints

Remain on your back with your legs outstretched. Clasp your hands just below your left knee and gently pull it toward your chest B, just as far as you can go. Hold for the count of five. You should feel a "pull" in the buttocks on the same side as the leg that you are working. Release the tension and gently bounce your knee toward your chest, then lower it, placing your foot back on the bed. Do five to 10 repetitions of this movement. Then repeat with the right leg.

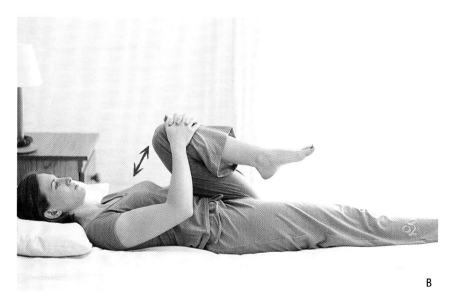

Mobilizing the lower joints in the vertebral column

Lie on your back, with your legs outstretched. Pull one knee to your chest C, hold it there, then pull the other knee up to your chest, too, so that you form a ball with your body D. Hold for the count of five, then release. You should feel a "pull" in both buttocks, or a slight stretch in your lower back. This stretch could be uncomfortable at first but should loosen up the more you do it. Do five to 10 repetitions.

Mobilizing the neural structures in the vertebral column

Lying on your back, pull both your knees towards your chest E. Hold them there and at the same time put your chin on your chest F. This should give you a good stretch right across your back. Hold for the count of five, then relax. Do five repetitions of this exercise. You should never experience sharp pain anywhere, but a good tight feeling is normal.

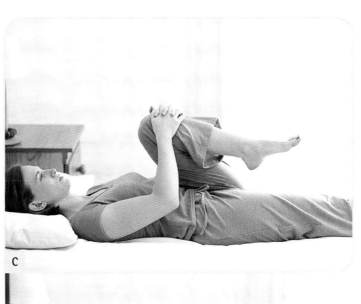

C

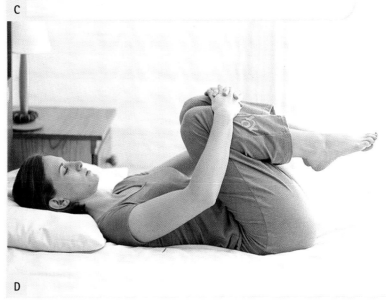

D

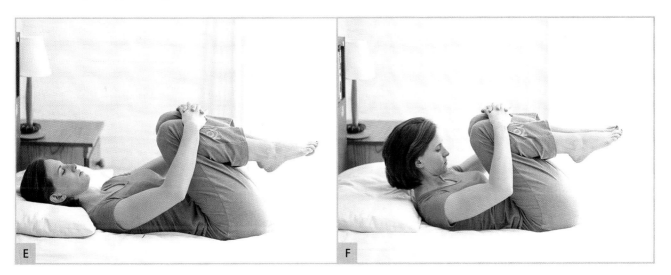

E

F

Mobilizing the back

This exercise mobilizes the back by encouraging it into its normal hollowing position while stretching the muscles in front of the vertebral column.

Lie face down on your stomach. Place your hands just under your shoulders, as if you are going to do a push-up A . Straighten your arms out, pushing your upper body up and backwards B , but keep your pelvis and legs on the bed. Hold for the count of five. This will hollow your back and loosen it in the opposite direction to the previous exercise. Do five repetitions of this exercise in a gentle, smooth manner. If the movement is stiff, then work only to the point of stiffness, not to the point of pain.

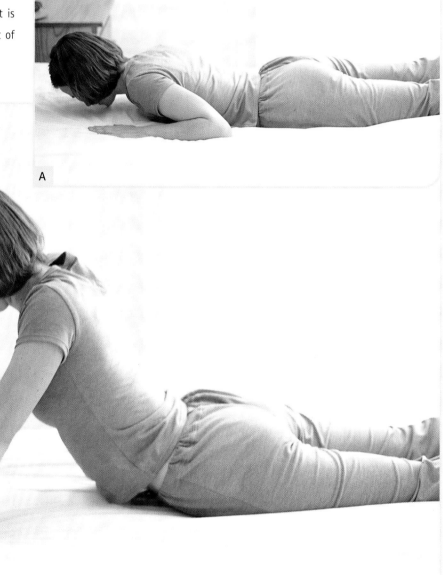

A

B

Mobilizing the neural structures in the leg

Lie on your back with your legs straight. Lift your left leg to form a 90-degree angle with your body C. Hold it there with your hands supporting the back of your knee, then straighten your leg out and flex your foot D until you feel a gentle "pull". Hold for the count of five, then bend the knee at 90 degrees again. Straighten the leg again, hold for the count of five, and release. You should feel the stretch in the back of your leg. It should not be too painful or cause you any acute pain in your back. Do 10 repetitions of this exercise. Then repeat with the right leg.

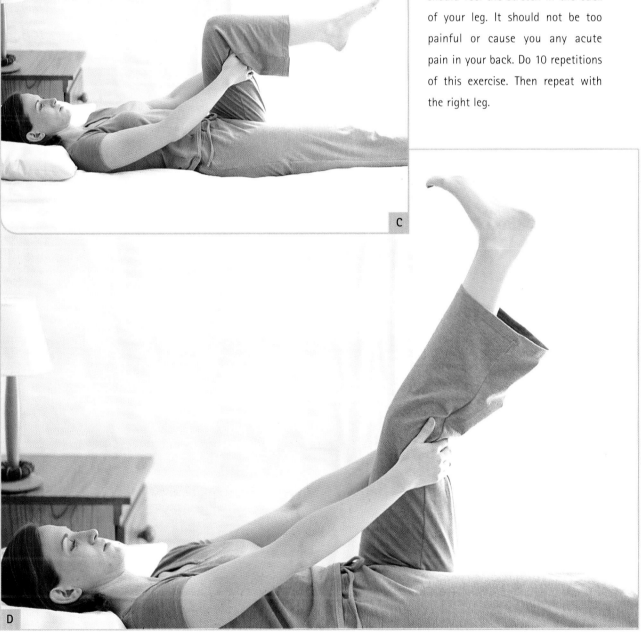

Stretching the muscles in your lower back

Lie on your back with your legs straight. Using both hands, pull your left knee up toward your chest A . Extend your left arm out horizontally to the left and, keeping your eyes trained on the left hand, use your other hand to pull your knee across your body toward the right side B . This movement will rotate your vertebral column. Hold for the count of 20, then relax. Do two repetitions on each side. You will feel the stretch in those areas where you are most stiff — it might be in the upper left part of your back, or the lower part, your buttocks or even in your arm.

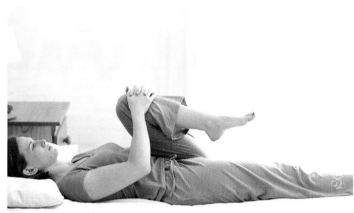

A

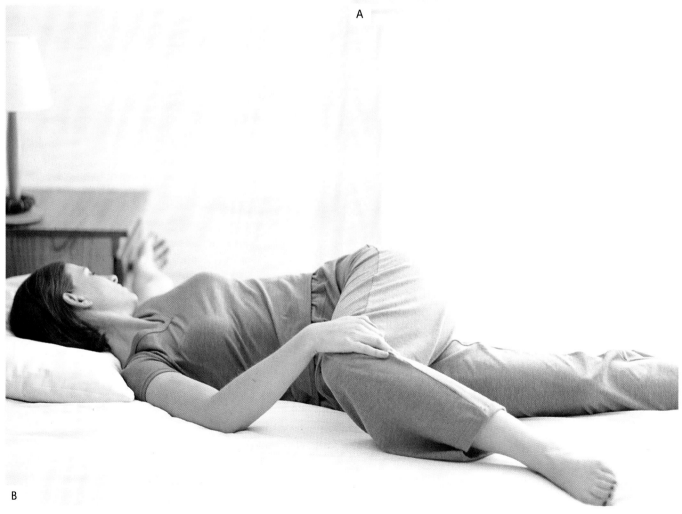

B

Stretching the muscles in your buttocks

Lie on your back with your legs straight. Bend your right leg slightly and place your right hand on your right knee A . Keeping your hand there, place your left hand on your right ankle and use both hands to pull the knee toward your left shoulder B . Hold the stretch for the count of 20, then relax. Do two repetitions of this movement toward the left, then alternate and pull the left leg toward the right shoulder. You should feel a "pull" in your buttocks as you stretch the deep gluteal muscle, the piriformis.

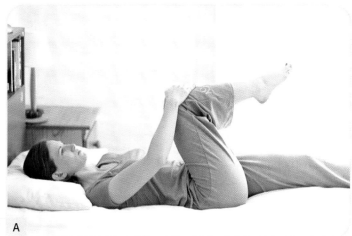

A

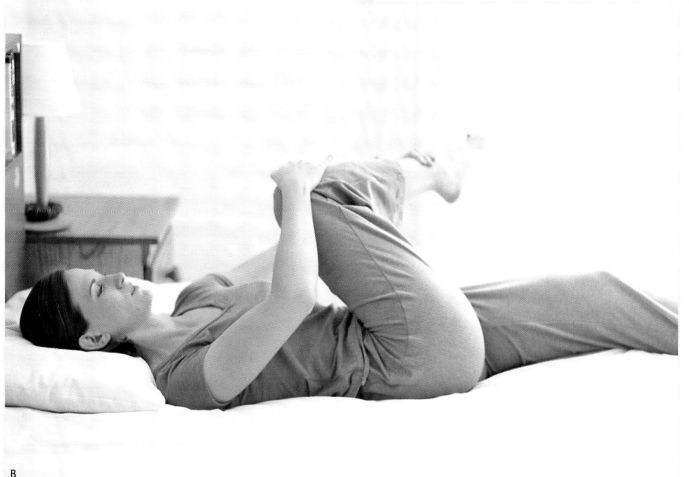

B

ACTIVATING YOUR STABILIZERS

Your stabilizers essentially consist of the transverse abdominus, all its supporting muscles and the thoraco-lumbar fascia. This stabilizing system forms a corset-like structure around the body, which serves to support the lower back. It is important that this system be activated before a movement begins so that your lower back can remain stable while the rest of your body moves. By preventing unnecessary movement of the lower back, you protect the vertebral column. Few people realize that it is largely the abdominal muscles that are responsible for this.

Your abdominal muscles support your lower back.

The importance of activating your stabilizers (contracting the transverse abdominus) cannot be stressed enough. The contraction should always be mild and controlled (about 20 percent of the full muscle effort) and be maintained throughout the movement. Make sure that you do the following exercises correctly, in the recommended sequence, and that you incorporate them into your daily routine. (Ensure that you are able to contract the transverse abdominus correctly before attempting any of the exercises in Chapter 3.)

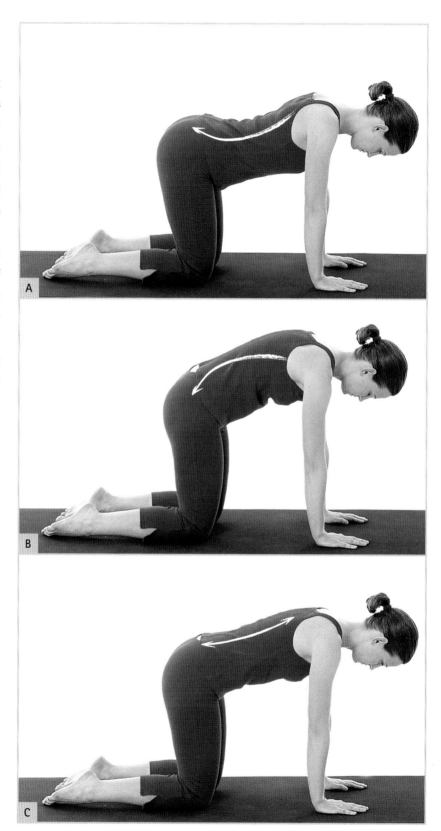

← Contracting the transverse abdominus

Correct activation of your abdominal stabilizers can seem quite complicated at first, but don't give up until you have tried it a few times.

Begin in the four-point kneeling position, hands and knees on the floor. Make a hollow with your back [A], then round it by tilting your pelvis [B] and settle into a neutral position at a midpoint between the two extremes [C]. This is the neutral position for your lower back.

Keeping your lower back fixed in this position, "drop" your stomach so that you feel it move closer to the floor. Next, pull the lower part of your stomach, the section below your navel, up toward your vertebral column in a gentle contraction. This will tighten your lower stomach muscles slightly. The stomach muscles above

WATCH OUT FOR THESE PROBLEM AREAS

- Don't move your back. Stay in the neutral position, i.e. the midpoint between an arched and hollow back.
- Don't pull your upper abdominals in under your chest.
- Don't stop breathing or use inhalation to pull your tummy in. Your ribcage should not move at all.

If you are doing any of the above while attempting this contraction then you are doing it incorrectly. Do not progress to the individual exercises until you get the isolated muscle contraction right. Don't despair — it takes some practice!

your navel should not move. If you have managed to contract your abdominal stabilizers correctly, hold for the count of 30, then relax. Do 10 repetitions of this exercise.

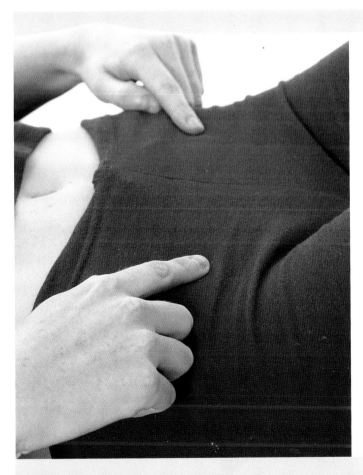

Just to make sure

For an alternative position to practice contracting the abdominal stabilizers, lie on your back with your knees slightly bent. Put your fingers on your pelvic bone (as shown) and slide them along the bone towards the middle of your abdomen to feel the tension of the muscle. It should be soft and relaxed. When you contract the transverse abdominus correctly, your navel should pull in and down and you should feel a slight tightening of the muscle under your fingers, pulling it flat. If you don't feel it, return to the four-point kneeling position and practice the contraction until you are sure you have got it right.

↓ Stabilizing your vertebral column while moving one leg

Lie on your back with your knees slightly bent, and contract the transverse abdominus (place your fingers on the pelvic bone, as described on p41, to make sure you are doing it correctly). With your stabilizers contracted, slide your left foot down on the floor until your leg is straightened out ⓐ, then bring it back to the starting position. While you are doing this you should concentrate on what your fingers are feeling. The pelvic bone should not move at all — if it moves, it means your lower back is moving as well, and this means that the stabilizers are not working hard enough (i.e. not correctly contracted).

The aim of this exercise is to train the stabilizing abdominal muscles to keep the vertebral column still while the leg is moving. If you find it difficult to tell whether you are doing the movement correctly, put your hand behind your back and make sure there is no movement against it during the exercise. Do five repetitions with each leg; progress until you can do 20 with each leg before you move on to the next exercise.

→ Using your stabilizers while standing

Stand upright, with your body as close to the ideal alignment (see p46) as possible ⓑ. Contract your stabilizers. Hold for the count of 20, breathing normally. If you can do this easily and are able to hold the contraction for the count of 30, then you can progress to walking.

First, try to walk just 10 paces keeping your stabilizers activated. If the transverse abdominus is correctly contracted, your lower back should not move. Progress to walking for a few minutes at a time. The ultimate aim is to do this every time you walk, making the activation of your stabilizers part of your daily life.

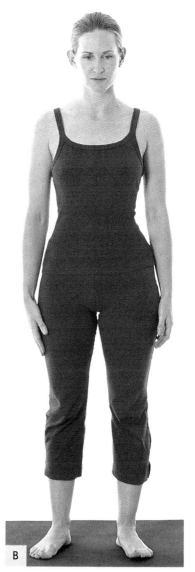

B

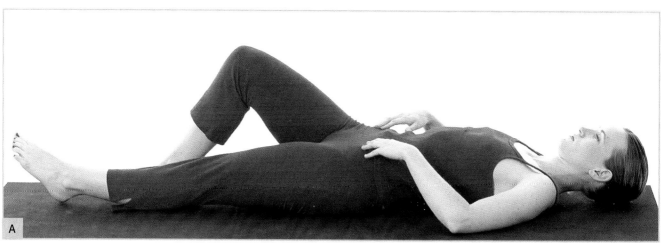

A

Using your stabilizers constantly

In the broadest sense, it is ideal to have your stabilizers active with every move that you make. Therefore, with every activity and/or exercise it is important that you first activate your stabilizers and then keep them correctly contracted throughout.

When lifting or picking up an object from the floor, it is imperative that you do not bend your back. To ensure you are able to maintain the correct posture you may need to strengthen your upper thigh muscles.

Start off with one leg placed slightly in front of the other A. Keep your posture in the ideal alignment and your stabilizers active. Bend both your knees B and go into a half-kneeling position, with one knee on the floor and the other bent at 90 degrees C. Return to the standing position and relax your stabilizers. Do five repetitions of this exercise. Repeat with the other leg.

If you struggle with this exercise, you may want to hold onto a chair at first. Do the exercise daily, however, and you will soon be able to do it without any support. The response elicited by this exercise should become automatic during all your lifting activities.

USE IT OR LOSE IT
- People who experience lower back problems don't use their stabilizers correctly.
- Your stabilizers have to be used correctly, i.e. correctly activated and in the correct sequence, to effectively support the lower back.
- Your abdominal stabilizers must be incorporated into your daily activity in order to provide maximum benefit.
- Correct use of your stabilizers contributes to improved posture and an ideal alignment.

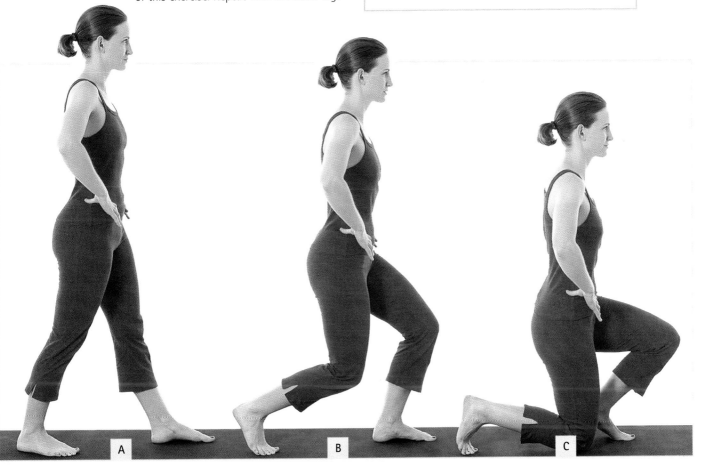

A   B   C

IMPROVING NEURAL MOBILITY

Our neural structures need to be kept mobile; only then will they allow the muscles to function more effectively. Neural mobility exercises are not common practice, which is unfortunate as they are extremely important for everyone. Sportsmen and women in particular will benefit from improved neural mobility, as well as individuals recovering from back operations (in this case, however, do not do these exercises without first consulting your doctor or therapist).

The following exercises are movements, not stretches. The aim is to move an area of your body in order to achieve a smooth, gliding motion of the nerve. You should feel a "pull" or tightness in the area you are working. Should you feel persistent "pins and needles", or experience pain during or after any of these exercises, consult your doctor.

Arm mobility exercises

⬇ Exercise 1

Stand up straight with your feet placed slightly apart. Keep your arms next to your body with your elbows straight and your arms turned outwards, wrist bent upward [A].

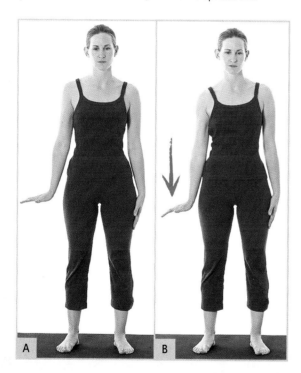

Keeping the rest of your body still, push your right hand down towards the floor [B]. You should feel a "pull" somewhere in the shoulder or along the arm. Return to the starting position. Do 10 repetitions of this movement. Then repeat with the left arm.

➡ Exercise 2

Stand in a door frame and place your hands on the inner frame to either side of you. Take a step forward, through the door [C], until you feel a "pull" in your shoulder area or arm. Return to the starting position. Do five repetitions of this movement (and five times a day for best results).

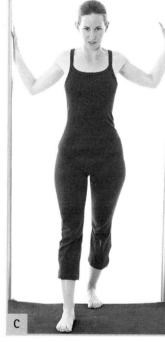

↘ Exercise 3

Standing upright, lift your right arm out sideways. Keep it straight, with the wrist turned up. Bring your left arm up and bend it at the elbow so that your left hand is against your head [D], with the wrist bent so that your hand is pointing towards your ear. Hold for the count of five, then repeat the movement with the other arm. Do 10 repetitions of this, alternating arms.

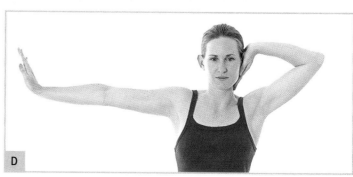

Leg mobility exercises

Lie on your back and, keeping your right leg straight and on the floor, lift your left leg, bending it at 90 degrees. Clasp your hands behind your knee and pull it gently towards your chest E . Next, straighten the leg until you feel a pull F , then release. Finally, straighten the left knee again, flex the foot up and down G , and release. Do 10 repetitions of each movement. Repeat with the right leg.

Neural mobility exercises for the full body

(**Please note:** this exercise should be done with utmost care, and only if you find the arm and leg neural mobility exercises reasonably easy.)

Sit with your legs straight out in front of you H (as an option you can press your feet flat against a wall, too). Keeping your head down, round your back as much as is comfortable I . Keep your knees straight and bend your neck further forward as you increase the arch. You should feel a "pulling" sensation in the back of the legs, but it should not be uncomfortable. Do not bend at the waist. Return to the starting position. Do five repetitions.

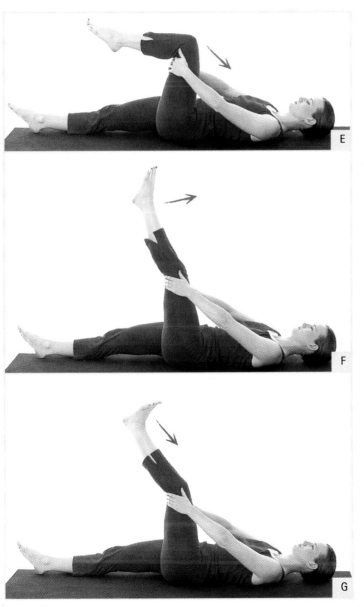

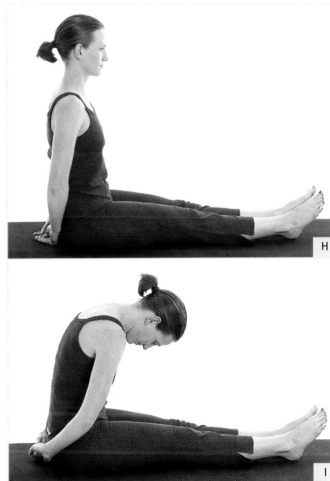

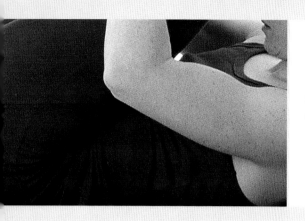

Analyzing Posture

Posture describes the way that you carry yourself. Every individual has different characteristics and a unique way of functioning and of keeping his or her body in alignment. Each posture uses and affects different structures in the back in a specific way, and some of these structures can cause lower back problems. Several postural patterns can be easily identified, and although it is sometimes impossible to correct postural problems totally, you can attempt to improve your posture by doing things correctly and by incorporating a few simple exercises into your daily routine.

THE IDEAL ALIGNMENT

If you look at the body in profile, you can draw a plumb (vertical) line that passes through specific structures to indicate an ideal alignment (see fig 1). In the case of good postural alignment, the line must:

- go through the ear
- go through the middle of the neck
- go through the middle of the waist
- lie slightly to the back of the middle of the hip joint
- lie slightly to the front of the middle of the knee joint
- lie just in front of the ankle joint

When the body is viewed from the back, the plumb line should traverse the head, the middle of the vertebral column (from top to bottom), the middle of the pelvis area, and end centrally positioned between the feet (see fig 2). This indicates that the weight distribution is even. If the line does not go through certain structures, it indicates the

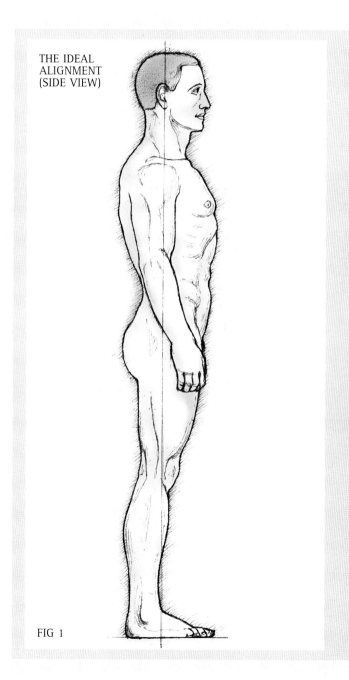

THE IDEAL
ALIGNMENT
(SIDE VIEW)

FIG 1

presence of an incorrect posture. The reason for so-called faulty posture is that the line of gravity does not cross the center of the joints. This indicates that there is:

- excessive muscle activity in the surrounding muscles to balance that joint against gravitational forces
- excessive soft tissue strain of that joint
- excessive compression of the cartilage in that joint.

Common problem areas in the spine are the "transition spots," or areas where the natural "S" curve changes direction (see fig 3). These include the point where the neck joins the base of the skull (the atlanto-occipital joint), where the neck joins the thorax (cervico-thoracic level), where the thorax becomes the lower back (thoraco-lumbar level) and where the spine joins the fixed pelvis (lumbo-sacral level). At these points the postural angle, or curve, is aggravated, causing greater strain on the related structures.

THE IDEAL
ALIGNMENT
(BACK VIEW)

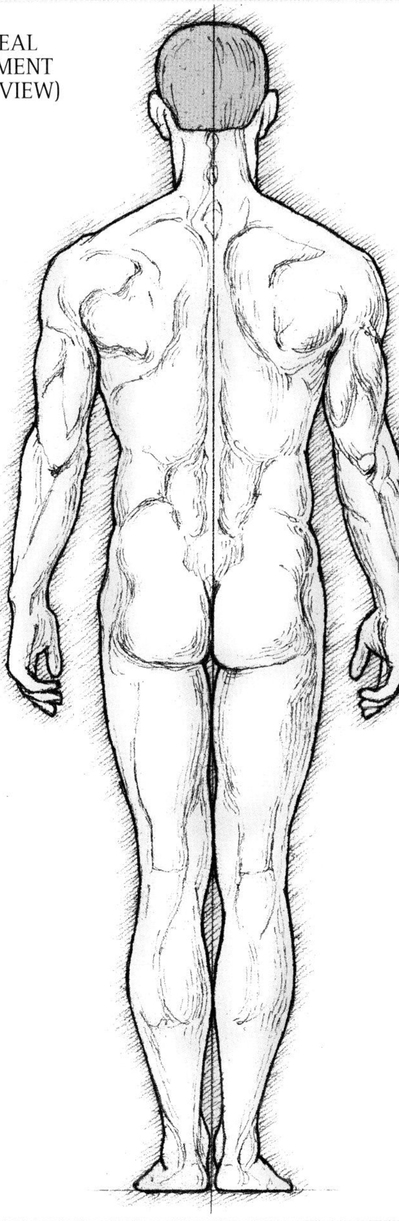

FIG 2

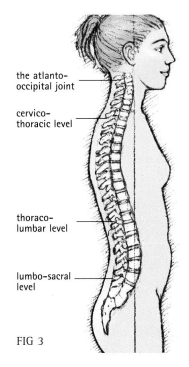

TRANSITION
SPOTS

the atlanto-
occipital joint

cervico-
thoracic level

thoraco-
lumbar level

lumbo-sacral
level

FIG 3

COMMON PROBLEM POSTURES

Having become familiar with the ideal alignment of the body you should easily be able to see where the following common faulty postures differ from the ideal. This information should help you to determine if you have an alignment problem. If you haven't had any problems with your back but find that you do have a slight alignment problem, it is recommended that you take note of the structures that could cause you trouble in the future and work towards improving your posture. Make use of the exercises listed on pp50–51.

By correcting your posture you will prevent excess strain on your vertebral column, helping to prevent back problems. If your postural problem is extreme, you may benefit from seeing a manual therapist who can evaluate your posture and work out an exercise program specifically suited to your needs.

Extreme kyphosis-lordosis posture

Extreme kyphosis-lordosis puts a lot of strain on the lower back (because of the increased hollowing of this area) and on the upper back (because of the increased rounding). The tension on the "transition spots" causes some structures to stiffen and others to loosen, affecting the proper function of joints and muscles.

Due to the increased curve in the vertebral column, the plumb line does not pass through the ideal alignment points (see fig 4). Instead, because the head is in a forward position, the line lies behind the ear. It lies to the back of the neck and lower back because of the increased hollowing of these points. Finally, because the trunk is so rounded, the line does not pass through the shoulder but in front of it, and as the pelvis is pushed out to the back, the line lies to the back of the hip and the knee and to the front of the ankle. (See chart on pp50–51 for affected areas.)

Flat-back posture

Although a lot of people think a straight spine indicates good posture, this is not always true. With flat-back posture the normal curves of the spine are straightened out, putting more strain on the back. The hips are pushed forward, the pelvis is pulled to the front, and the knees bend further back than normal, all of which puts more strain on these joints (see fig 5). (See chart on pp50–51 for affected areas.)

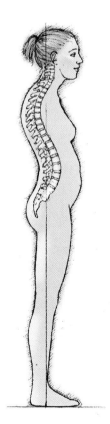

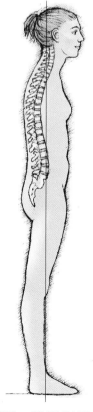

FIG 4: EXTREME KYPHOSIS-
LORDOSIS POSTURE

FIG 5: FLAT-BACK POSTURE

HIGH HEELS

When you wear high-heeled shoes, your center of gravity is altered. Normally, your center of gravity should be just in front of your ankle joint. When you raise your heel, you shift your center of gravity forward to the ball of your foot. To maintain balance, you then automatically hollow your back more, so as not to fall forward. These changes in your spine place more stress on the joints.

The sway-back posture

In the "sway-back" type of posture the head is even further forward than in the flat-back posture (see fig 6). The trunk area is rounded towards the back, the lower back is slightly rounded, instead of being hollow, and the hips are much further forward than in an ideal alignment, forcing the knees further back so that the person can still keep his or her balance. With the hips pushed forward and the back at an angle, the individual with this type of posture can look like he or she is constantly leaning or swaying backwards, hence the name. (See chart on pp50–51 for affected areas.)

Scoliosis

Spinal scoliosis is a lateral "S"-shaped curve of the spine that is easily identified when the person is viewed from behind. Unlike the other postural alignments, scoliosis can be a congenital abnormality; however, it can also present itself due to prolonged bad habits, for example, carrying a school backpack on only one shoulder or incorrect posture in standing. The scoliosis curvature can be either to the left or to the right (fig 7 illustrates a left curve) and can occur anywhere in the vertebral column, however, it generally affects more than one point of the spine. For example, if the primary curve (left curve) is in the lower back, a secondary curve will occur higher up the spine to compensate for the lower one. In fact, the rest of the body adjusts in order to achieve balance: the head tilts slightly to the right, the right shoulder drops while the left sits slightly higher, and the pelvis drops on the left, remaining higher on the right.

Although in some cases the vertebrae and intervertebral discs can be affected, people with scoliosis often do not experience pain at the curved area. The problems usually occur in the areas that have had to compensate — there can be pain in the neck, around the area of the shoulder blade, in the back at waist level and in the lower back. Manual therapy may help relieve the pain experienced in extreme cases. It is important to note that some forms of genetic scoliosis cannot be corrected and in these cases the joint should simply be kept mobile and the muscles strong enough to protect the back.

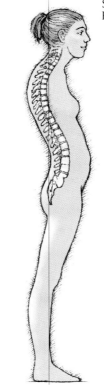

SWAY-BACK POSTURE

FIG 6

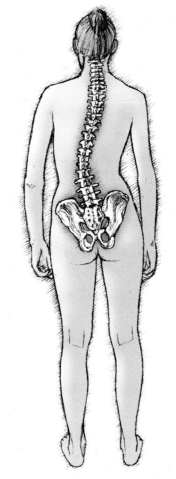

SCOLIOSIS

FIG 7

TYPE OF POSTURE	AREAS OF WEAKNESS	RELEVANT EXERCISES
1. Extreme kyphosis-lordosis (fig 4, p58)	• The front neck muscles • The scapula stabilizing muscles • The upper back muscles • The abdominal muscles • The gluteus • The hamstrings	Exercise 5 (p60) Exercise 7 (p61) Exercise 4.1 (p59) Exercise 1 (all) (pp52–56) Exercise 6 (p60) Exercise 2 (p57)
2. Flat-back (fig 5, p48)	• The front neck muscles • The scapula stabilizing muscles • The abdominal muscles • The quadriceps (muscles in front of the thigh) • The hip flexors (in front of the hip)	Exercise 5 (p60) Exercise 7 (p61) Exercise 1 (pp52–56) Exercise 3 (p58) Exercise 3.2 (p58)
3. Sway-back (fig 6, p49)	• The front neck muscles • The scapula stabilizing muscles • The lower back muscles • The abdominal muscles • The quadriceps • The hip flexors	Exercise 5 (p60) Exercise 7 (p61) Exercise 4.2 (p59) Exercise 1 (pp52–56) Exercise 3 (p58) Exercise 3.2 (p58)
4. Scoliosis (left curve) (fig 7, p49)	• The left trunk muscles • The right hip abductors (the muscles lifting the right leg outwards) • The left adductors (the inner thigh muscles)	**Please note:** Because scoliosis is a complicated postural problem and characteristics may vary from person to person, it is best to see a manual therapist who will work out a specific program tailored to suit your needs.

AREAS OF TIGHTENING

RELEVANT EXERCISES

- The back neck muscles
- The pectoralis and the structures in front of the shoulders
- The lower back muscles
- The hip flexors

Exercise 12 (pp60–61)
Exercise 11.1 (p64)

Exercise 11 (pp64–65)
Exercise 8 (p62)

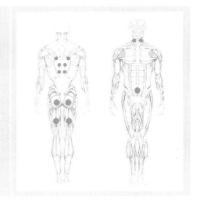

- The back neck muscles
- The pectoralis and the structures in front of the shoulders
- The gluteus
- The hamstrings

Exercise 12 (pp66–67)
Exercise 11.1 (p64)

Exercise 10 (p64)
Exercise 9 (p63)

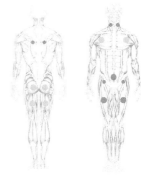

- The back neck muscles
- The pectoralis and the structures in front of the shoulders
- The gluteus
- The hamstrings

Exercise 12 (pp66–67)
Exercise 11.1 (p64)

Exercise 10 (p64)
Exercise 9 (p63)

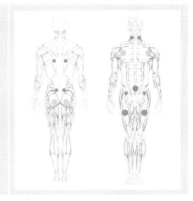

- The right trunk muscles
- The left hip abductors (the muscles lifting the left hip outwards)
- The right adductors (the inner thigh muscles)

Please note: Because scoliosis is a complicated postural problem and characteristics may vary from person to person, it is best to see a manual therapist who will work out a specific program tailored to suit your needs.

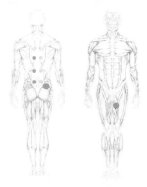

51

EXERCISES TO IMPROVE POSTURE

As already identified, different postures lead to weakness in certain structures and tightness in others. If you do nothing to counteract this, you will inevitably experience back problems. A few simple exercises will help strengthen and/or loosen the relevant muscles and ligaments. To determine which exercises will benefit you, use the information already presented in this chapter to identify your posture type and the structures that could be affected. Refer to the panel on pp50—51 to identify the exercises that will balance the effects of your posture. These exercises are outlined below — by working them into your daily routine you will be less likely to develop back problems.

1. Strengthening the abdominal muscles

The transverse abdominus is the most important stabilizing muscle when it comes to the lower back; it should be the first muscle to contract before any movement takes place, and the last to relax. Unfortunately, most of us are unaware of this and as a result, neglect to use it or strengthen it. Several important exercises specific to this purpose have already been outlined in Chapter 3, however, the following exercises, relating more specifically to posture, will also help you in this regard.

Exercise 1.1

Begin in the four-point kneeling position, hands and knees on the floor. Make a hollow with your back, then round it, and settle into a neutral position at a mid-point between the two extremes. Hold this position for the duration of this exercise (and remember to contract your abdominal stabilizers before beginning each movement).

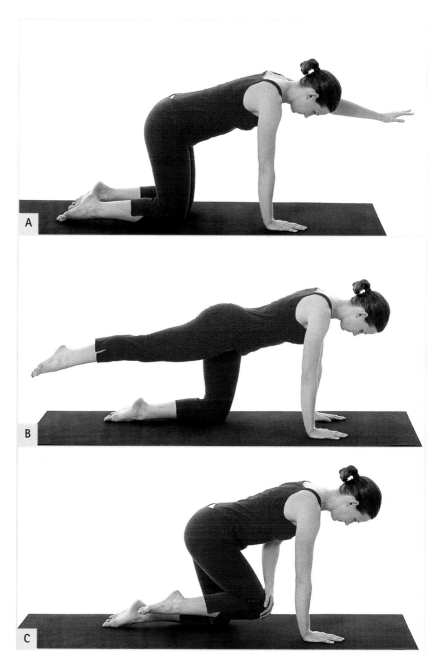

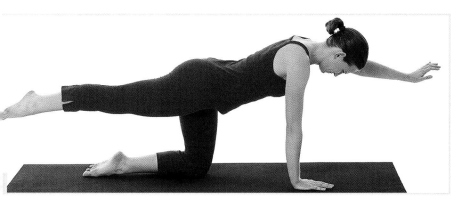

Keeping your neck in line with your spine, lift your left arm up, straighten it out in front of you A, and lower it back into the resting position. Do 10 repetitions. Repeat with the right arm.

Next, lift the right leg up, extend it out behind you B, and lower it back into the resting position. Do 10 repetitions. Repeat with the left leg.

Again with your neck in line with your spine, touch the right knee with the left hand C, then return to the resting position. Do 10 repetitions.

Next, touch the left knee with your right hand, and return to the resting position. Do 10 repetitions.

Making sure you maintain the neutral position, lift and straighten the left arm and the right leg simultaneously D. Hold for the count of five. Return to the resting position. Repeat 10 times. Then repeat with the right arm and left leg.

Exercise 1.2

Lie on your back with your knees slightly bent and your feet resting on the floor E. Find a neutral position by hollowing and rounding your back and settling into a midpoint between the two extremes. (Ensure that you correctly contract your stabilizers while you are doing this exercise.)

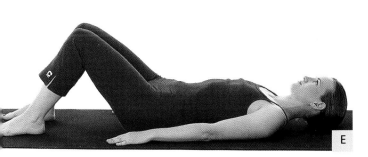

Raise your left arm and extend it above your shoulder. Straighten your right leg simultaneously F. Hold for the count of five, then bring your arm and leg back to the starting position. Do five repetitions. There should be no movement in the lower back while doing this.

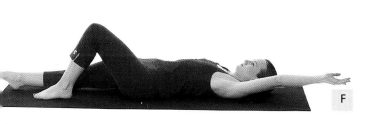

Next, raise your right arm and straighten your left leg simultaneously G, hold for the count of five and return to the starting position. Do five repetitions. This exercise will mimic the walking pattern and prepare you for keeping your lower back still while walking.

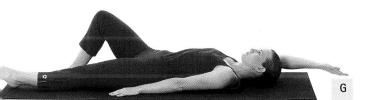

Exercise 1.3

Lie on your back. Bend your knees slightly, and with your feet slightly spread apart, raise your hips off the floor, keeping your shoulders and head on the mat A . Contract your abdominal muscles and hold. This is the starting position for the next sequence of exercises.

Raise your left knee and bring it slightly toward your chest, until it makes a 90-degree angle with your body B .

Hold for the count of five and return to the starting position. Do 10 repetitions. Then repeat with the right leg.

With hips still raised, extend the left leg C , hold for the count of five, and bring it back to the starting position. Keep your balance, and your abdominal muscles contracted. You should not move your lower back at all. Do 10 repetitions. Repeat from the beginning with the right leg.

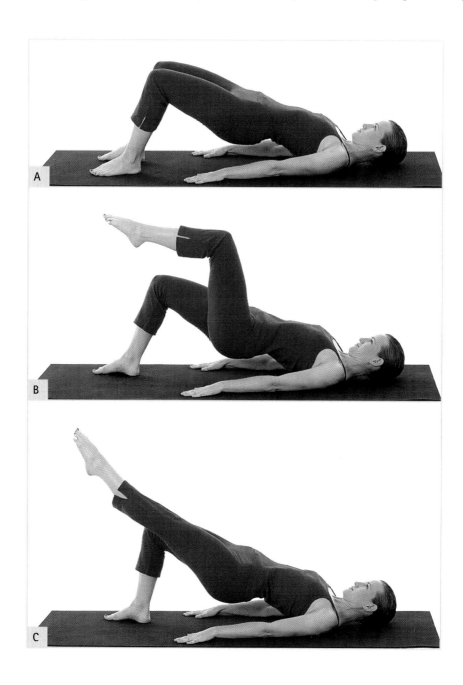

Exercise 1.4

Get into position on your left side; your head, hips and ankles should all be in line with your shoulders. You can support your head on your outstretched arm, while your right (top) arm rests lightly on the floor in front of you. Bend your left (bottom) leg at the knee to give you more support. Contract your abdominal muscles.

Lift your right (top) leg in line with your body. Make small circles using the whole leg D. Do this rotating clockwise five times and counterclockwise another five.

Next, make big circles with your whole leg E. Rotate clockwise five times and counterclockwise another five.

Remember that your pelvis and back should not move at all during this exercise. Roll over to lie on your right-hand side. Repeat exercise 1.4 with the left leg.

Exercise 1.5

Return to the starting position on your left side, only this time support yourself on your left elbow, bent at a 90-degree angle, and keep your right arm in front of you F. Place your right (top) leg on the floor just in front of your left (bottom) leg. Contract your abdominal muscles and lift your hips off the floor G. You should feel a strong contraction in your lower back and abdominal area.

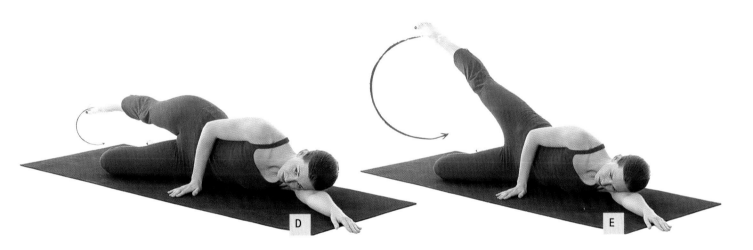

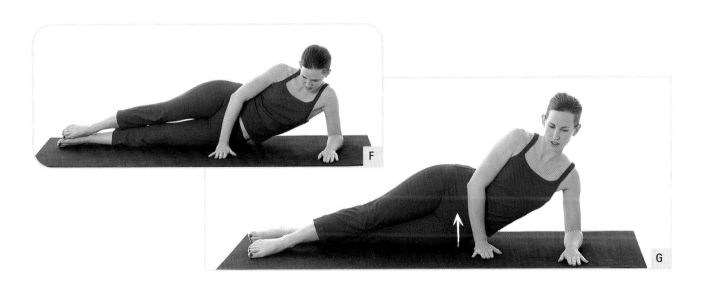

Keep your hips off the floor for the count of five and slowly bring them back down. Repeat this five times. Then change over and do five repetitions on the right side.

For a more advanced version of this exercise, keep your feet in line with your body, one leg on top of the other A. Push down on your arms and lift your hips off the floor B. Remember to contract your abdominal muscles and keep your lower back in the neutral position.

Again, keep your hips off the floor for the count of five and slowly bring them back down. Repeat, five times on each side. You can progress and hold for a count of 10, for 10 repetitions.

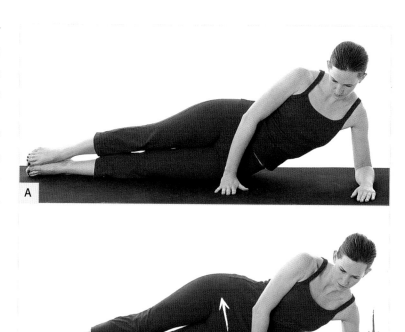

Exercise 1.6

Lie flat on your stomach with your toes turned in. Contract your abdominal muscles, then push up onto your forearms C. Make sure you keep your head in line with your body and your elbows directly under your shoulders.

Push down on your forearms and lift your hips (and your knees) off the floor D. Hold this position for the count of five, drop your pelvis and relax. Do five repetitions. Progress to 10, holding for the count of 10.

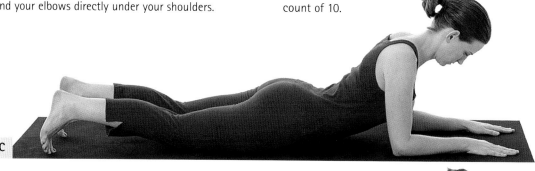

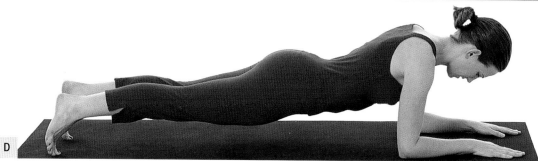

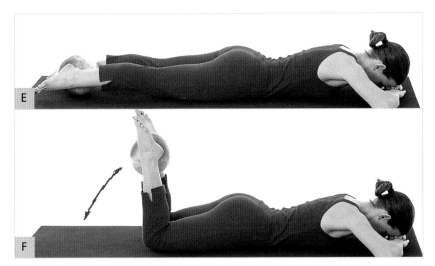

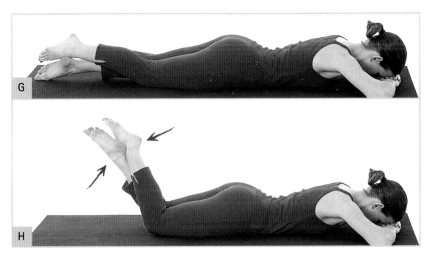

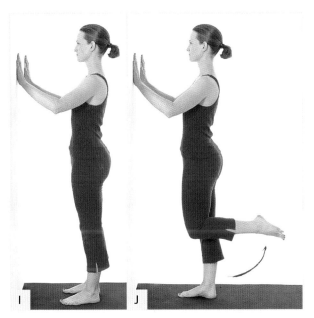

2. Strengthening the hamstrings

Exercise 2.1

Lie flat on your stomach, rest your head on your hands, and pinch a small ball (e.g. football) between your feet E. Make sure that you do not hollow your lower back during this exercise.

Bend your knees, keeping the ball pinched between your feet F. Hold for the count of five. Then slowly straighten your knees again, lowering your legs without dropping the ball. Do 20 repetitions of this exercise.

Exercise 2.2

Still lying on your stomach, cross your legs at the ankle, right over left G. Slowly bend your left knee back H. The right leg resting on the left leg will offer some resistance — it should be just enough to make it difficult without stopping the movement. Do 10 repetitions. Change legs, bending the right knee back with the left leg offering resistance. Do 10 repetitions.

Exercise 2.3

Stand facing a wall. Rest your hands lightly in front of you for support I. Bend your left knee back, at an angle of 90 degrees J. Hold for the count of five, then slowly straighten it out again. Do 20 repetitions of this exercise. Repeat with the right leg. (Note: you can add weights to your ankles to make your muscles work harder.)

3. Strengthening the quadriceps

Exercise 3.1

Stand upright with your back in the neutral position, your hands resting on your hips and your right leg slightly in front of your left [A]. Contract your abdominal muscles and bend your knees slowly for the count of three, lowering your back knee towards the ground [B]. Then slowly return to the starting position for the count of three. Do 10 repetitions of this exercise. Switch legs and repeat

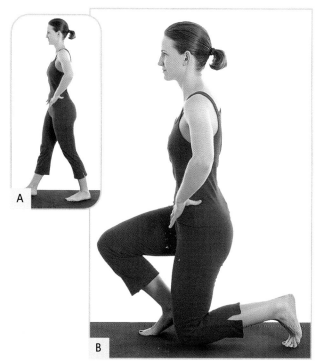

10 times. If you find this exercise difficult, you may want to use a chair or table initially for support.

Exercise 3.2

Stand with your back against a wall, with your feet hips-width apart and about 8in (20cm) away from the wall. Make sure your lower back, your head and your shoulder blades are touching the wall [C]. Keep your lower back in the neutral position and contract your abdominal muscles.

Bend your knees to about a 90-degree angle [D]. Lowering your hips, hold this position for the count of five, then slowly come up for the count of five. Do 10 repetitions.

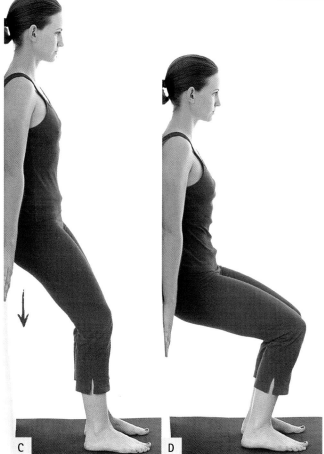

4. Strengthening the back muscles

Lie on your stomach, with only your upper body resting on a flat surface, e.g. a table E. Be sure that the table will support your weight! Keep your lower back in the neutral position and contract your abdominal muscles. Bend your arms at the elbow and place them on either side of your head.

Exercise 4.1 – Upper back muscles

With your hands lightly resting on your temples, raise your head and shoulders slightly off the surface F. Hold for the count of five. This should not hollow your back; if it does, you have moved too far. Do 10 repetitions.

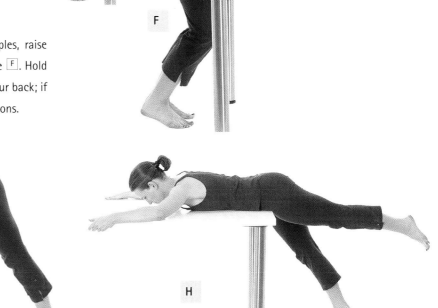

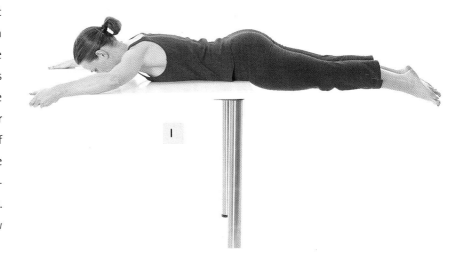

Exercise 4.2 – Lower back muscles

Still on your stomach, straighten your legs out slightly behind you until you are resting on your toes G. Keeping your lower back in the neutral position and your abdominal muscles contracted, hold on to both sides of the table and lift one leg until it is line with your upper body H. Hold this position for the count of five, then relax. Do 5 repetitions. For a more advanced movement, lift both legs simultaneously I and again hold for the count of five. Be careful not to lift too far as this will hollow your back unnaturally and lead to problems.

59

5. Strengthening the neck muscles (front)

Lie on your back and keep your eyes on the ceiling A. Pull your chin toward you, as if you are nodding B, without lifting your head off the mat. Do 10 repetitions of this subtle movement. You should feel your head sliding up and down on the mat with this exercise.

If you feel ready to progress to a more advanced version of this exercise, lift your head slightly off the mat with each nodding movement, but keep your chin tucked in all the way. And so the sequence should be: tuck your chin in, lift your head, hold for the count of five, then return to the starting position. Do five repetitions of this movement.

6. Strengthening the gluteus muscles

Lie on your left side, with your knees bent at a 45-degree angle. Support your head on your outstretched arm and keep your top hand in front of your body for additional support C. Contract your abdominal stabilizers and raise your right knee D. Make sure you keep your top foot resting on the bottom foot and that you don't move your pelvis. Hold your knee in the raised position for the count of five, then bring it back down to the resting position. Do 20 repetitions of this movement. Then repeat on your right side, raising your left leg.

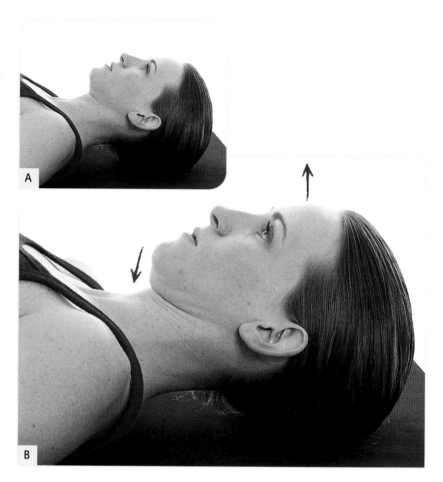

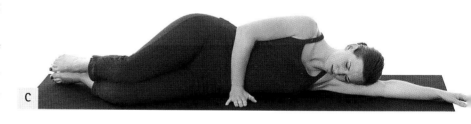

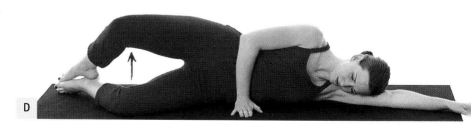

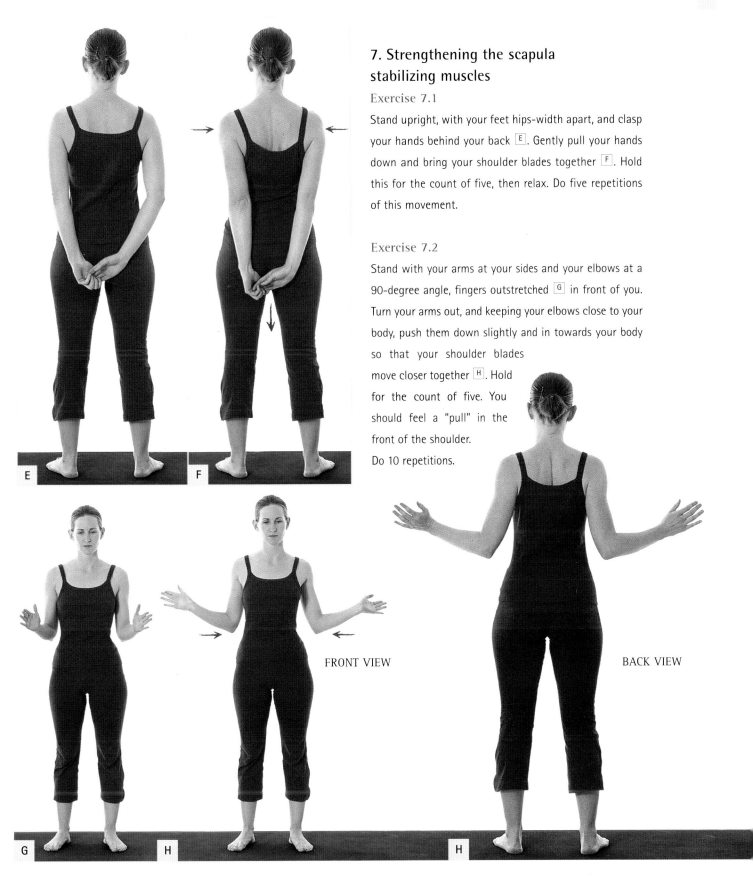

7. Strengthening the scapula stabilizing muscles

Exercise 7.1

Stand upright, with your feet hips-width apart, and clasp your hands behind your back E. Gently pull your hands down and bring your shoulder blades together F. Hold this for the count of five, then relax. Do five repetitions of this movement.

Exercise 7.2

Stand with your arms at your sides and your elbows at a 90-degree angle, fingers outstretched G in front of you. Turn your arms out, and keeping your elbows close to your body, push them down slightly and in towards your body so that your shoulder blades move closer together H. Hold for the count of five. You should feel a "pull" in the front of the shoulder. Do 10 repetitions.

FRONT VIEW

BACK VIEW

8. Stretching the hip flexors

Exercise 8.1

Stand with your left leg on the floor and your right leg bent at a 90-degree angle, resting on a bench or low chair A. Keep your lower back in the neutral position and contract your abdominal muscles.

Lean forward until you feel a pull in the left leg B in the groin area. Hold it for the count of 20. Do two repetitions of this stretch. Switch legs and repeat.

Exercise 8.2

Step into a lunge with your left leg forward, and lower yourself until your right (back) knee is resting on the ground. Lightly rest your hands just above your left knee and lean forward, putting your weight on the left foot C. You should feel a "pulling" sensation in the groin area of your right (back) leg. Hold it for the count of 20. Switch legs and repeat.

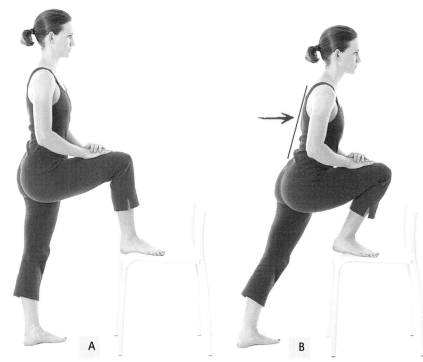

A

B

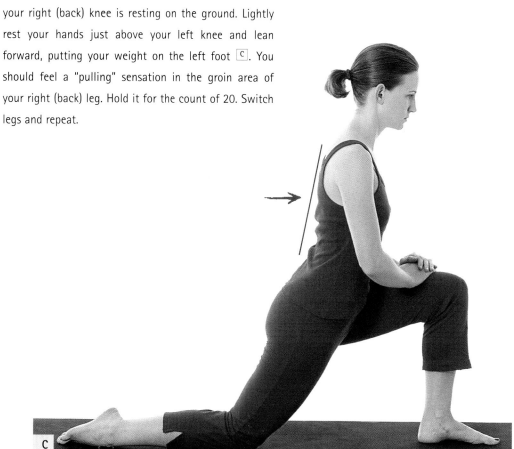

C

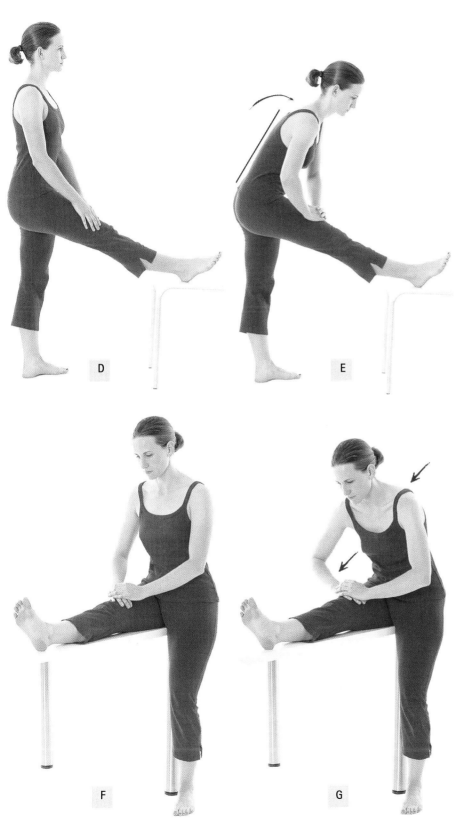

D

E

F

G

9. Stretching the hamstrings

Exercise 9.1

Stand with your left leg on the floor and your right leg outstretched, the heel on a higher surface, e.g. a chair ⌑D⌑. Rest your hands lightly just above your knee and bend forward at the hips ⌑E⌑ making sure you do not round your back. You should feel a "pull" in the back of your right thigh. Hold for the count of 20. Do two repetitions. Switch legs and repeat.

Exercise 9.2

Sit on the edge of a firm bed or low table with your right leg straight out in front of you and your left foot resting on the floor ⌑F⌑. Gently rest your hands just above the right knee. Bend forward until you feel the "pull" in the back of your straightened (left) leg ⌑G⌑. Hold this stretch for the count of 20. Do two repetitions. Switch legs and repeat.

(**Please note**: you should not feel any pain in your lower back with either of these hamstring stretches. If you do, it would be wise to consult a professional.)

10. Stretching the gluteus muscles

Lie on your back and pull your left knee up towards your chest. Put your left hand on your knee and wrap your right hand around your left ankle A.

Pull your left knee towards the opposite shoulder B with the right hand supporting the movement at the ankle. Hold for the count of 20. You should feel a "pulling" sensation in the buttock area. Do two repetitions of this stretch. Switch legs and repeat.

11. Stretching the back muscles

Exercise 11.1

Lie on your back. Bend your right knee at 90 degrees and rest your left hand on the knee joint C. Extend your right arm out above your head to incorporate the pectoralis (chest muscles). Pull your right leg across your body and turn your head towards your extended right hand D. You should feel a "pull" on the right side of your body. Hold this stretch for the count of 20, then relax. Do two repetitions of this movement. Switch sides and repeat.

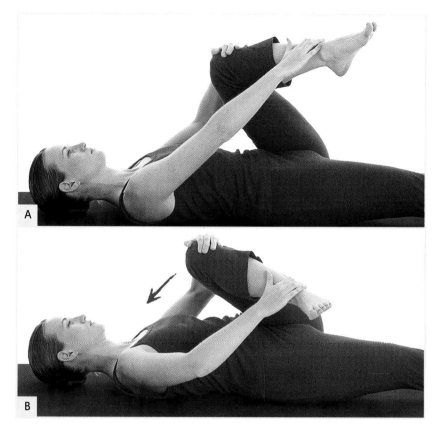

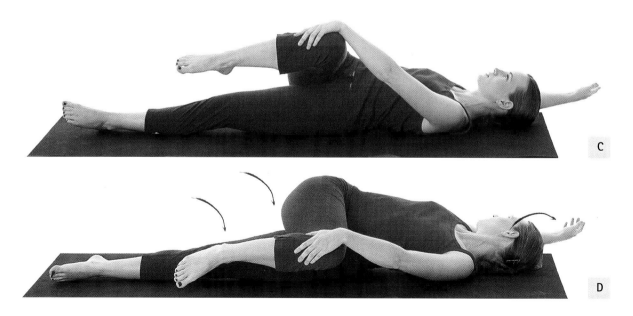

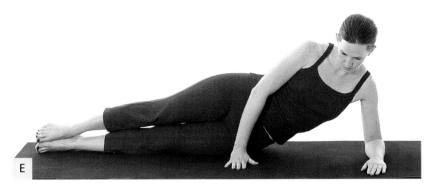

E

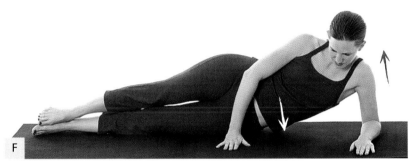

F

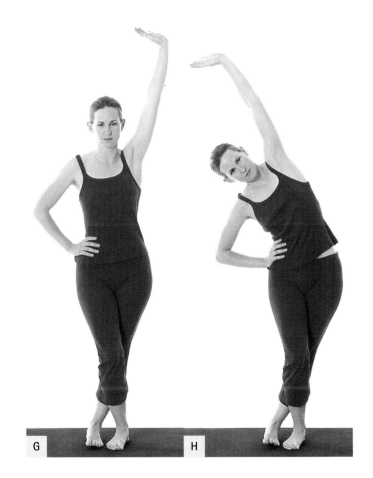

G   H

Exercise 11.2

Lie on your left side and support yourself on your elbow, bent at a 90-degree angle. Keep your right hand in front of your body for additional support E. Breathe in, then on the out breath push your left side down into the floor F. You should feel a "pull" on the left side of your lower back. Hold this stretch for the count of 10, then relax. Do five repetitions. Switch sides and repeat.

Exercise 11.3

Stand upright, with your right leg crossed over your left. Place your right hand on your waist for support G. Lift your left arm above your head and stretch it over to the right, bending your upper body in the same direction H. You should feel a "pull" on the left side of your lower back. Hold this stretch for the count of 20. Do two repetitions.

Switch your legs around, left in front of right, and repeat.

You can do this exercise with your back against a wall, if needed for balance. Alternatively, if bending to the right, you can put your left hand on a table. The important thing is to allow the spine to bend sideways.

12. Stretching the neck muscles

Exercise 12.1

Sit up straight on a straight-backed chair. Place your left hand on the right side of your head A and gently stretch your neck towards your left shoulder B. You should feel a "pull" on the right side of your neck. With your right hand, hold onto your chair to keep your right shoulder down. Hold for the count of 20. Do two repetitions. Switch around and repeat on the other side. (**Please note**: you should not feel any discomfort in your neck on the side towards which you are stretching.)

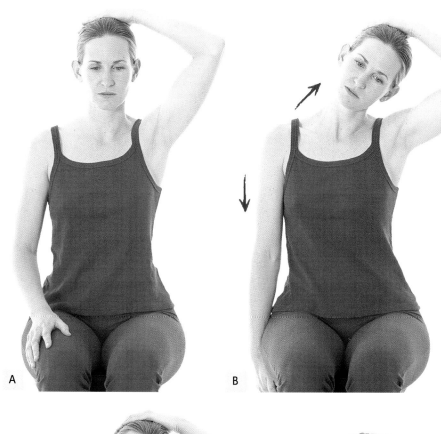

A

B

Exercise 12.2

Sit upright, with your right hand holding onto your seat. Place your left hand on the right side of your head and pull it gently towards the left shoulder C, then tilt your head up towards the right. Gently stretch your head towards your left shoulder D. You should feel the stretch on the right side of your neck. Hold for the count of 20. Do two repetitions. Switch arms and repeat on the other side.

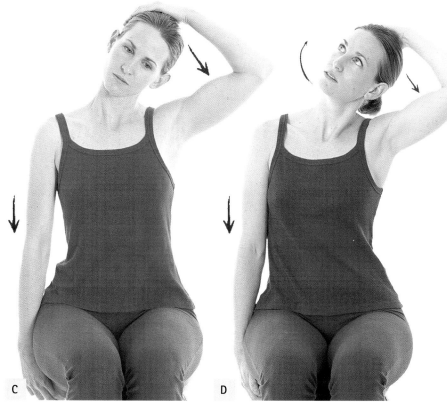

C

D

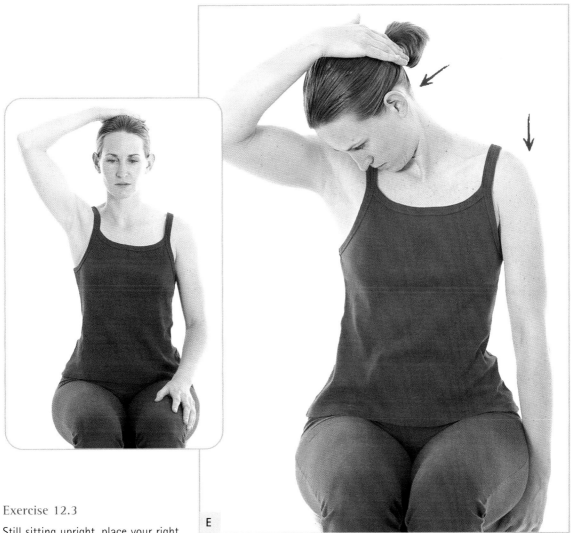

E

Exercise 12.3

Still sitting upright, place your right hand on the left side of your head and tilt your head down and to the right so that you are looking under your armpit E . Apply pressure with your hand and gently press your head down. Hold onto your chair with your left hand to keep your shoulder down. You should feel a "pull" on the left side of your neck. Hold for the count of 20. Do two repetitions of this stretch. Switch arms and repeat on the other side.

Please note: these exercises are particularly beneficial for individuals who work at a computer and they can be carried out during breaks. People who suffer from chronic cervical headaches should also do these exercises — they loosen the structures in the neck which are the cause of pain. The stretches work well in the shower, with hot water running over the muscles that are being stretched.

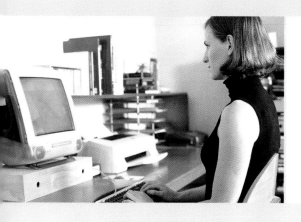

Achieving Good Posture

By doing certain things in an incorrect position, you will definitely put more strain on the joints, ligaments and muscles in your back. Long-standing bad habits, in particular, can lead to problems over time. To avoid this, it is important to be aware of the correct way of performing day-to-day activities. This chapter provides an overview of the recommended postures for performing even those activities we think come naturally, such as sleeping.

POSTURE IN STANDING

When standing, you need to retain your lower back and neck's "hollowing" (lordosis) while your upper back keeps its "rounding" (kyphosis). These curves should not be straightened out nor excessively pronounced. Your back in the ideal alignment described in Chapter 4 (see p46) would constitute the ideal posture when standing. When this neutral position is maintained, the joints are under less strain and the ligament and muscle activity necessary to maintain the position of the spine is limited to a minimum.

NEUTRAL POSITION

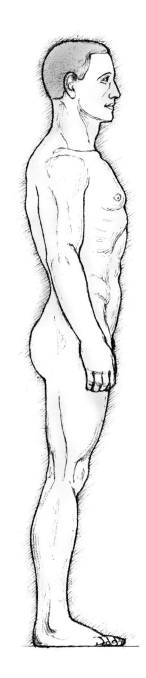

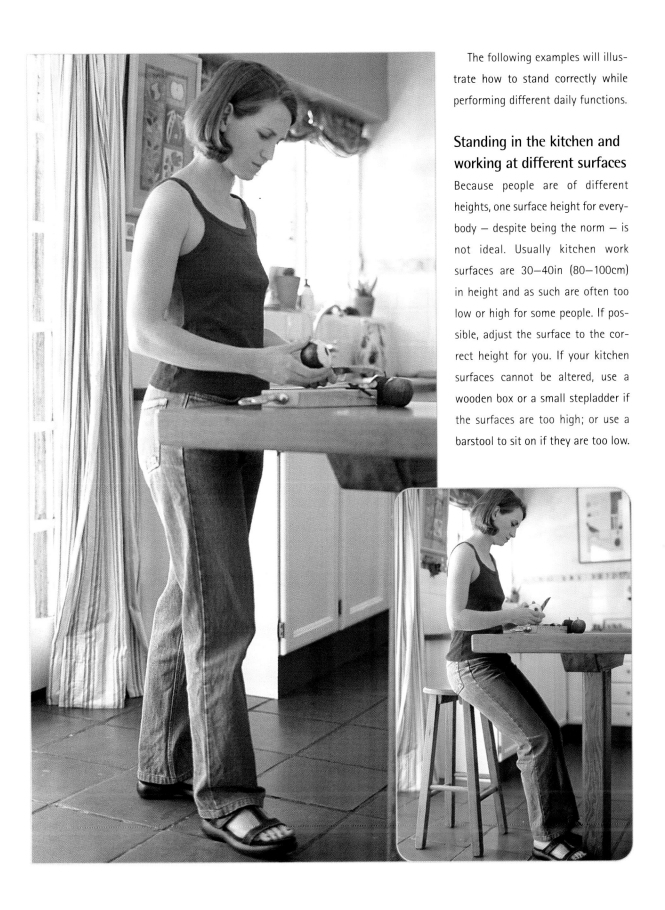

The following examples will illustrate how to stand correctly while performing different daily functions.

Standing in the kitchen and working at different surfaces

Because people are of different heights, one surface height for everybody — despite being the norm — is not ideal. Usually kitchen work surfaces are 30—40in (80—100cm) in height and as such are often too low or high for some people. If possible, adjust the surface to the correct height for you. If your kitchen surfaces cannot be altered, use a wooden box or a small stepladder if the surfaces are too high; or use a barstool to sit on if they are too low.

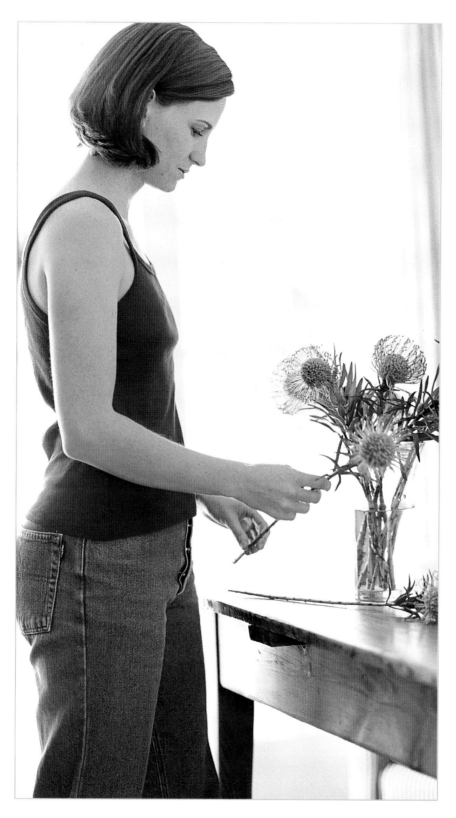

If you are doing light work (e.g. peeling fruit), the work surface should be at elbow height. If you are doing more strenuous work, e.g. kneading dough, you need to work at a lower surface, one that is at the level of your hands if your elbows are bent at about 45 degrees. Remember to take into account the object that you are working with. For example, if you are arranging flowers, the height of the vase should be considered and it is this that should be at elbow height, not the surface it rests on (see picture).

The way you stand in front of a surface is also important. Stand close so that you don't need to lean over too far to reach things. If the surface is wide and you need to reach in deep, it is best to stand with one leg in front of the other. This way, when you reach out, you can move your weight onto the front foot, leaning forward without having to bend your back.

If you are standing for long periods of time, it is important to take short breaks. Stop what you are doing. If you have been leaning forward, bend your back in the opposite direction for a few seconds (see opposite). Doing this every few minutes will take some of the strain off your back while you are working, preventing it from becoming stiff and painful.

Standing while ironing

Ironing is often a long and tedious chore. Very few people enjoy it because it can be tiring for the lower back. To take some of the strain off your lower back, try standing with one foot on a surface that is slightly higher, i.e. the cross bar under the ironing board or a small box. With one leg in front of the other, you can also change your weight between the two and avoid bending your back in order to reach the furthest corner of the ironing board. It is important to take short breaks and stretch your back backwards a few times to relieve the strain. Do this before your back starts feeling tired, at least every 20–30 minutes.

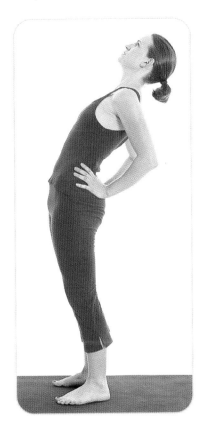

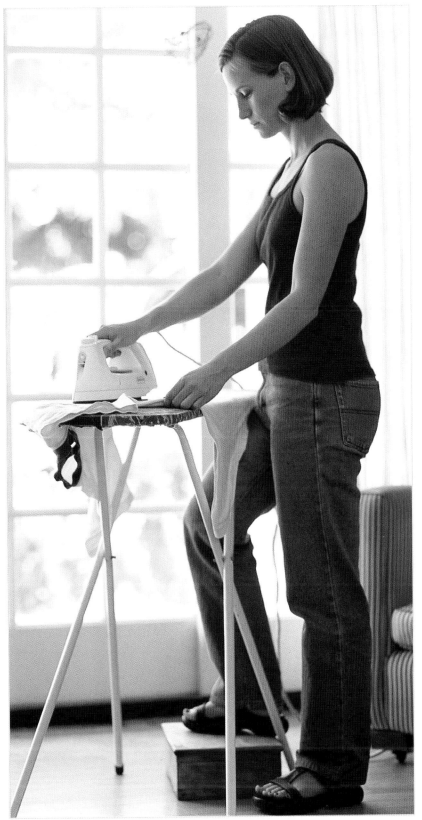

Standing while vacuuming or sweeping

When vacuuming or sweeping, stand with your legs one in front of the other so that you can distribute your weight evenly. As your upper body moves forward and backward with the broom or vacuum handle, you will be able to keep your lower back still by shifting your weight from one leg to the other. Keep your abdominal stabilizers contracted and your lower back in the neutral position. To avoid bending too far forward, ensure that your broom and/or vacuum cleaner has a long handle. For very heavy cleaning, make sure that you alternate jobs. Don't wash all the walls at once; do something else and then come back to the job. Short and frequent breaks will protect your back and relieve unnecessary strain.

Standing and doing woodwork

Woodwork can be a strenuous activity, drawing on physical strength and heavy body movements. It is important to have a surface to work on that is lower than your elbow height, i.e. the height of your hands if your elbows are bent at a 45-degree angle. Not only will you have a better view of what you are doing, you will also be able to put some weight behind your movements. Take the thickness of the wood you are working with into consideration as it might alter the height of the surface. To ensure that your balancing muscles are not overworked, provide a wide support base by standing with your feet well apart. Take short breaks, moving your back in the opposite direction to the one you have been working in.

Standing and playing a musical instrument

Playing a musical instrument often means spending hours on your feet. Long periods in one position are not good for your back; the joints become less flexible and the muscles tend to tighten. Again, it is important to take short breaks and stretch your back, neck and arms. This

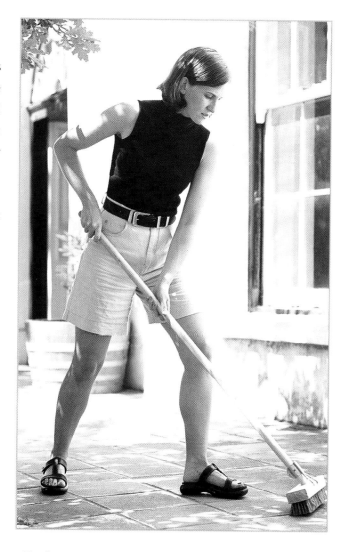

will relieve some of the tension in these areas. You don't have to do all these stretches during the same break, rather focus on something different during each one. A few stretches every 20–30 minutes is ideal.

Make sure you are standing up straight even though you sometimes have the instrument on one side. Try and maintain the neutral position of the ideal alignment while practicing; leaning across or sideways for long periods of time will lead to a painful stiffness in your back. Sustaining one position for a long period of time may shorten some muscles and weaken others. Stretching before and after practicing will be of great benefit, just as it is for athletes.

Standing in a train or on a bus

The surface you might stand on in a train or on a bus, though solid, is constantly moving. The vehicle stops and starts, often with a jerk. To prevent your back having to absorb any jerking movements, stand with one leg in front of the other in the direction of the movement. This will enable you to keep your back still and distribute your weight between both legs to compensate for unexpected movements. Standing in the neutral position, taking equal weight on both feet, keeps your stabilizing muscles contracted and protects your lower back from unexpected movements. Holding on to something will make you even more stable.

Children carrying backpacks

It is important to have a good backpack that offers adequate support for the lower back. A child's school backpack should have wide shoulder straps and should not hang down too low, it should not be too heavy and

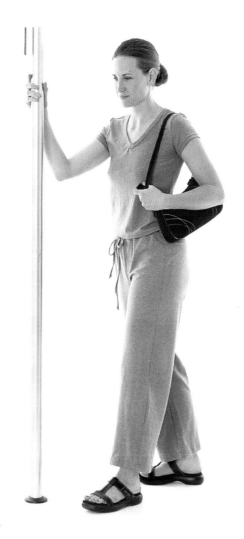

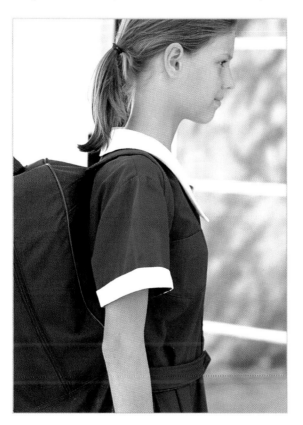

should feel equally weighted on the shoulders. Children often use the correct bags but carry them incorrectly. The straps, for example, should be worn on both shoulders allowing the weight of the bag to be evenly distributed. Many children use only one support strap, hanging all the weight on one shoulder. The back is forced to bend toward one side, compressing the joints and potentially leading to back problems. Wearing a bag on the same side for a long period of time may cause you to develop a skew back (scoliosis), which could also cause back pain.

Carry your bag correctly at all times and keep your stabilizers contracted to protect your back while doing so. There are good and bad products on the market so choose your backpack carefully.

POSTURE IN SITTING

Sitting puts a lot of strain on the lower back — it causes a 50 percent higher compression on the lower back discs than standing does (*see chart on p24, different loads in different positions*). Think about where you work or what you like to do for entertainment. You'll probably find that most of your daily activity — traveling on a bus or train, working at a desk, watching television, eating — involves sitting down. Because so many of us spend long periods of time in a seated position, we need to make certain that it is the correct one.

To ensure you are sitting correctly make sure that:

1   Your feet are supported on the floor.
2   Your knees are bent at a 90-degree angle.
3   Your hips are at the same height or slightly higher than your knees.
4   Your back is fully supported — especially in the hollow curve.
5   You sit far back into your seat.
6   Your head and shoulders are in line with your hips.
7   Your abdominal stabilizers are contracted.

CORRECT SITTING POSTURE

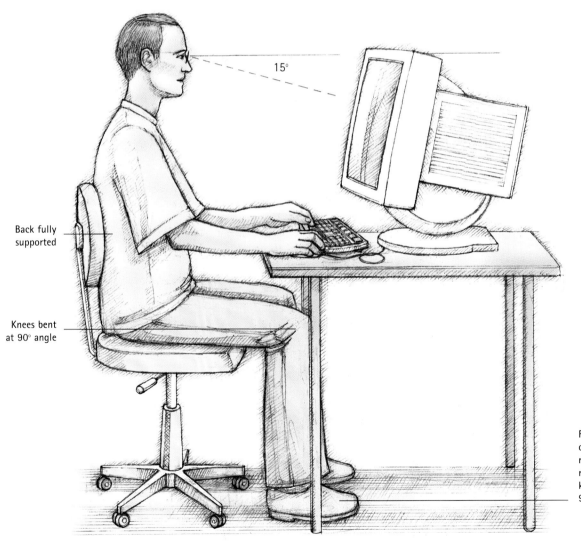

15°

Back fully
supported

Knees bent
at 90° angle

Feet supported
on the floor, or
raised on a box, if
needed, so that the
knees remain at a
90° angle.

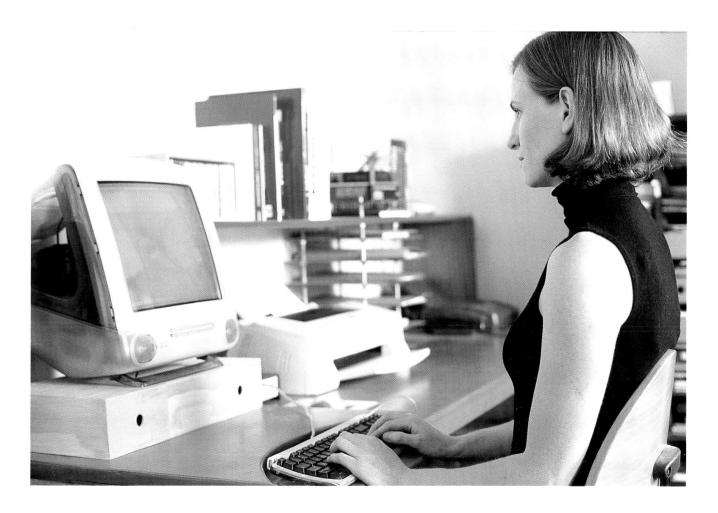

Sitting in front of the computer

It is important, when sitting in front of a computer, to check the height of your keyboard and your screen. In the seated position, your work surface should ideally be at elbow height. So should your keyboard. Your computer screen should be positioned straight in front of you, not to one side. It should be 15 degrees lower than the height of your eyes and about an arm's length away from you. Lighting should be adequate and the screen should be in focus.

Take short breaks regularly while working at the computer.

If you do a lot of typing, you should consider getting a stand to hold documents. Placed adjacent — and at the same height — to the screen, the stand will limit straining movements, such as looking up and down repeatedly. A good wrist pad and armrests are also recommended. If you have problems with your eyes, consider getting a bigger screen so that you can see more clearly without having to poke your chin forward. Similarly, if you wear bifocal lenses, avoid tilting your head back to look through the bottom of your glasses as this will put strain on your neck.

One tends to sit in front of the computer for long periods of time, forgetting about posture and not checking whether one is actually comfortable. Take a short break every 20–30 minutes. During these breaks move your neck from side to side and turn your back from left to right — this will help prevent strain on the back.

Have you got a good chair?

A good chair can contribute to good posture in sitting. The following characteristics are important:

- You should be able to adjust its height to suit your height and proportions as well as the level of your desk.
- It must be able to swivel, so that your body does not have to turn from left to right all the time.
- It must support the hollow part of your lower back.
- It must have armrests that are at the height of your elbows, when your arms are bent at 90 degrees.
- It must be the right height for the surface at which you are sitting, minimizing the amount of time you will have to bend down or lift your arms excessively to do your work.
- It must have a soft but firm cushion.
  Because we are all unique, of different shapes and sizes, one chair will not be correct for all of us. If you find your chair is not giving you adequate support, you should, for example, choose to make use of a small cushion to keep your back in the neutral position.

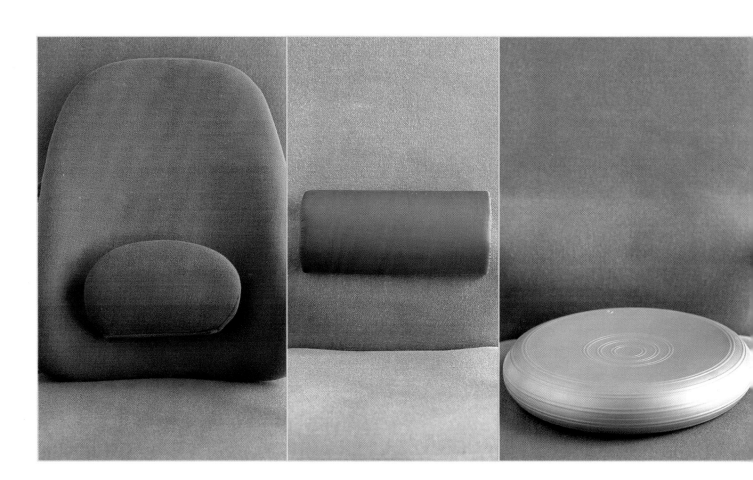

↑ Additional back rest with adjustable pillows. This cushion should sit in the hollow of your back to help it maintain its normal lordotic curve.

↑ An adjustable single pillow — which can be attached to most office chairs — serves to maintain the lower back's natural curve.

↑ This cushion is known as an air pillow. It provides an unstable surface and sitting on it forces you to activate your stabilizers.

Sitting and watching television or reading

The chairs or couches in your living room will most likely be soft and comfortable, and while you may start out sitting upright, as time goes by you will inevitably slide further into a "lounging" position. By sliding down the chair or couch you cause an excessive rounding of your back, and maintaining this position for a few hours subjects it to additional strain. By observing a few simple guidelines, it is possible to

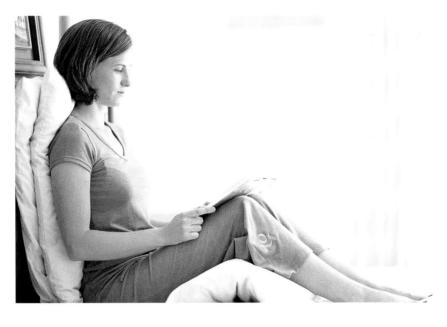

sit correctly for extended periods of time. Make sure that when you first sit down you settle right into the back of the chair, with your back in the neutral position. The principles discussed previously for

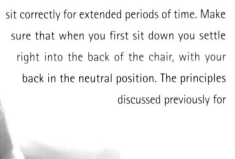

correct sitting posture (see p74) also apply when watching television. The height of the television should be neither too high nor too low — you should be able to keep your head in the neutral position while watching. Make sure that your chair is positioned in front of the screen so that you do not have to crane your neck to see the picture.

Lying in front of the television, be it on the couch or in bed, is often a problem: you tend to prop your head up with a few cushions, placing strain on the neck. If this is your favorite position for watching television or reading, try to keep your neck in the neutral position by sitting up a bit. You may even want to consider elevating the position of your television. (Many hospitals mount television screens on the ceiling so that patients can lie in a neutral position and still see the screen comfortably — if you can create the same effect, it will be much better for your back.)

Taking a break every now and then is also important; standing up and moving around is always good for your back. Maybe next time, you can volunteer to make the run to the kitchen!

Are you sitting correctly in front of the television?

Sitting and breast-feeding

Breastfeeding mothers often sit in one position for long periods of time, concerned about the baby and therefore not quite relaxed. It is important to sit in the neutral position, in a chair that offers good support, e.g. an armrest for your arm. Keeping your arm up with the baby lying in it tends to make you hitch your shoulder up and pull your back to that side. This puts a lot of strain on your upper back and your neck. You should put enough pillows under your arm so that your shoulder and arm can relax totally with the baby lying in the crook. It is important to breast-feed on both sides during one session as this will avoid excessive strain to one side.

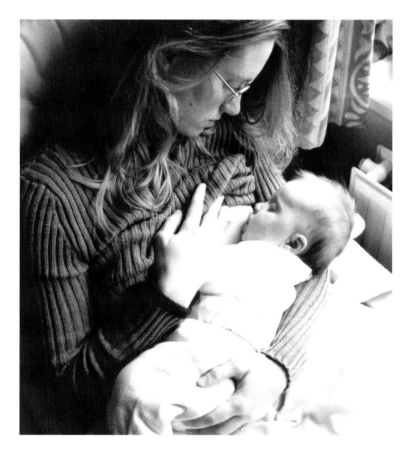

Sitting in and getting out of a car

Sitting in a car, sometimes for hours, is another position that many people have to cope with each day. Sitting for long periods of time, combined with the vibration of the vehicle, affects the discs of your lower back. This applies particularly to truck drivers, as the vibrations they experience are more vigorous and they often spend days behind the wheel.

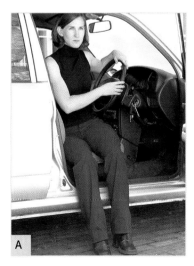

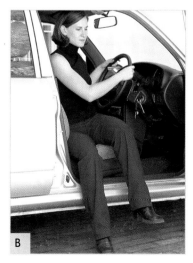

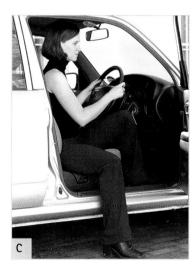

Getting in and out of a vehicle could be a source of strain. When getting into a car, lower yourself into the seat, but keep your feet on the ground A (see previous page). Swivel your pelvis and place one leg inside the car, then the second B + C . Try not to turn your back on its own; instead move your back and your legs at the same time. You will find this easier if your abdominal stabilizers are contracted. (When getting out, place one leg on the ground, then the second, before standing up. This will prevent an awkward rotation of your back, which happens when you stand with one leg in and one leg out of the car.)

Once in the car, the basics of the correct sitting posture, as described at the beginning of this chapter, are again important D . In addition, you should maintain a good distance from the pedals. Your knees should be slightly bent, so that it is comfortable to step on the pedals without having to straighten your leg completely. You should sit right into the back of the seat and maintain the neutral position for your lower back. Your shoulders should be in line with your lower back, and your head in line with your shoulders. Your hands should be in the "ten-to-two" position E and your elbows bent comfortably at about 45 degrees. When stopped at a traffic light, loosen your neck by moving it from left to right and stretching it gently from side to side by lowering your head toward your shoulders. On long trips, stop regularly (more often than to just fill up with gas) to give your back a break and stretch it in the opposite direction.

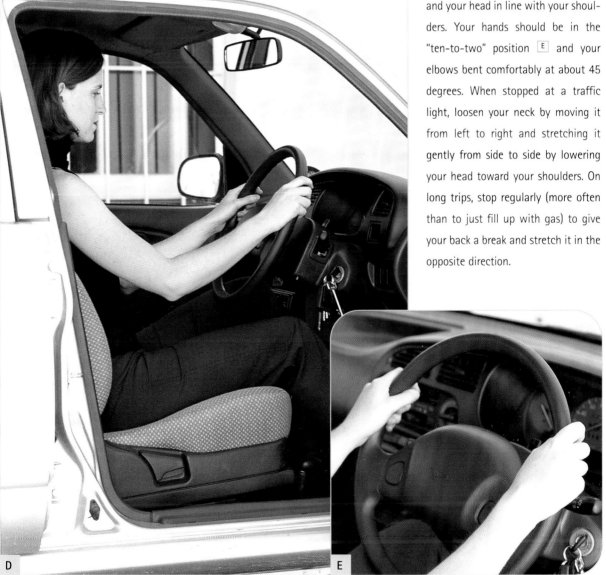

D

E

SLEEPING POSITIONS

While you are sleeping, your muscles relax completely and as a result your vertebral column loses the support of its active stabilizers. Because you are likely to spend six to eight hours in a specific position, it is vital that you try to maintain the neutral position while sleeping. If you lie with a rounded back, in the fetal position for example, your vertebral column will be stretched for hours; if you have too few or too many pillows, your neck will either be stretched or compressed for hours — all these factors could lead to problems over time.

Start off with a good mattress. Your mattress should be soft but firm and not have any holes or indentations. A mattress that is too soft and not supported on a firm base will not allow you to maintain the neutral position: your back and pelvis (the body's heaviest points when lying down) will make a permanent indentation and the mattress will no longer offer adequate support for your back.

The best position for your lower back is on your side as it allows you to maintain the neutral position. You can support your top leg with a pillow to keep your pelvis from rotating your lower back A.

Lying on your back is not a bad second option. If you experience discomfort in your lower back in this position, place a pillow under your knees B to help ease some of the strain caused by the pull of the hip flexors and hamstrings.

Sleeping on your stomach (prone position) C will not put undue strain on your lower back as long as you have a good firm mattress. It is advisable to place a pillow underneath your hips or your stomach D to prevent excessive hollowing. The prone position does put some

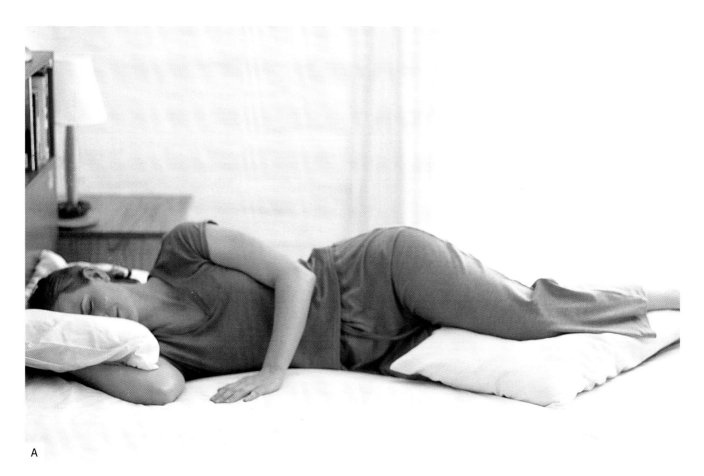

A

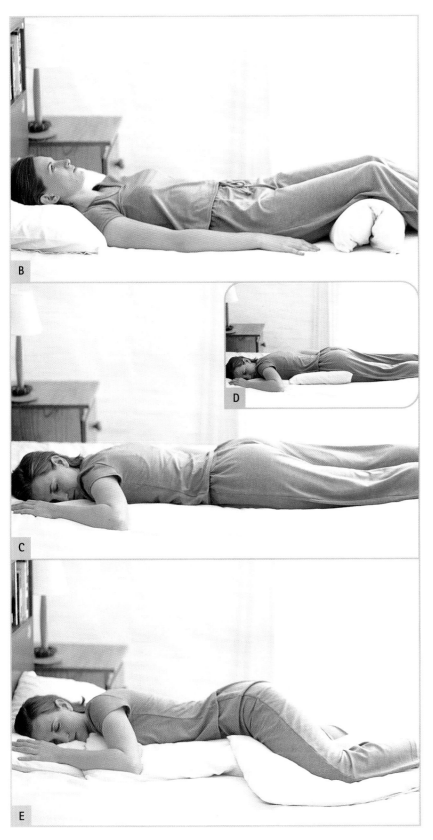

B

C

D

E

strain on your neck because it is forced to turn to the side. If you like sleeping on your stomach, try to turn slightly so that you are half on your stomach and half on your side. Place a pillow in front of and under your chest, and another one between your legs for comfort E.

As already evident, pillows are an important aid for posture when sleeping. Your head pillow should be just the right height to keep the neck in the neutral position and not bend it forward or backward. It is important to make sure that your shoulders are not on your pillow as it is only your neck and head that will benefit from support. You will need more height in your pillows when you sleep on your side than when you sleep on your back. (The distance from your shoulder to your neck when lying on your side is greater than the distance from the mattress to the back of your neck when lying on your back.)

It is difficult to recommend a standard number of pillows, or types, as pillows all vary in height and thickness. However, a pillow that can mold around your neck usually works well, e.g. a soft feather pillow. Specially designed pillows are only suitable if your neck is exactly the same as the one the pillow was designed for. If at all possible, it is best to try a pillow out before you purchase it.

LIFTING OBJECTS

Lifting and picking up objects puts a lot of strain on your lower back, especially when doing it repetitively. Lifting things correctly will take a bit more time but will save your back from painful injuries.

Remember to take small breaks and bend backwards often if lifting repetitively; also try to alternate lifting with other jobs. This will give the discs and muscles in your lower back time to recover from the increased strain

Some of the basic principles to consider when lifting an object are:

- Keep your back in the neutral position.
- Stand with one leg in front of the other in order to widen your base A.
- Keep your abdominal stabilizers active.
- Bend your knees, not your back B.
- Test the weight of the object before you lift it C.
- Keep the object close to your body D.
- Don't turn your back while lifting, rather move your feet and walk around to put objects down next to you.
- When lifting with another person, make sure you agree on when to lift — a simple "one, two, three" or "one, two, three, lift" can make a huge difference to help you correctly coordinate.

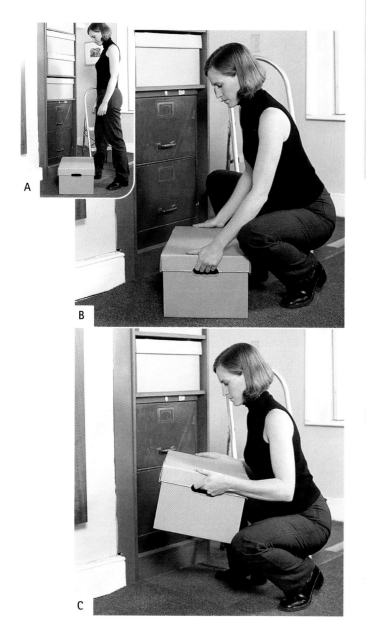

A

B

C

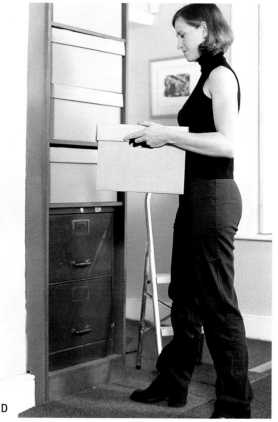

D

that has been put on them. Never think that because you are performing a task the whole day you are well equipped for the job. If your work involves repetitive lifting it is important that you train your body and keep fit. For heavy lifting, strengthen your quadriceps and your abdominal stabilizers so that you can work through the day without getting too tired. (see exercises in Chapter 4).

If you need to reach an object that is on a top shelf, for example, don't strain your back by reaching and juggling the weight above your shoulders. Rather make use of a small, sturdy box or step ladder, remove the object from the surface at eye level [A] and keep it close to your body [B] before setting it down.

If the object is too heavy, be wise and seek assistance! Don't first try to do it by yourself – this is too often the cause of injury. If you just need to move an object, e.g. a piece of furniture, sit down next to it, put your feet against it and push. Your thigh muscles are strong and made to take weight and they will save your lower back in this instance.

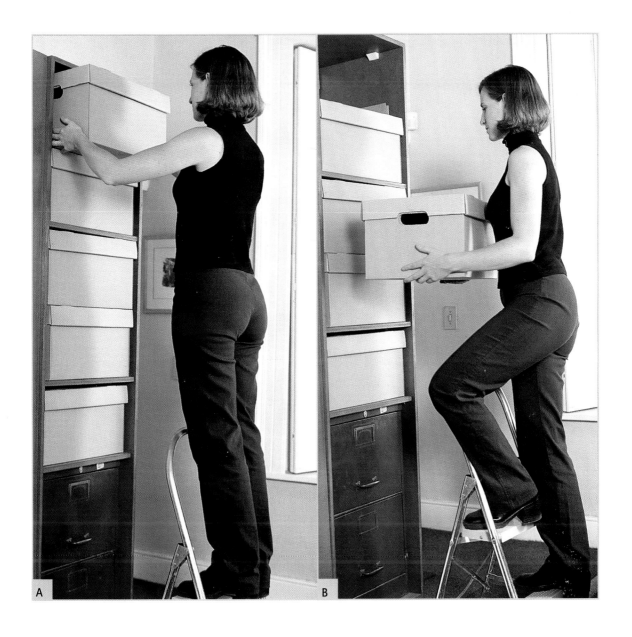

A   B

Carrying and picking up children

The principles for picking up objects also apply when picking up children. Resist the temptation to simply lean over and lift. Instead, with your feet placed slightly apart, bend your knees into a squat that will bring you closer to the level of the child A . Wrap one arm around the child's body and use the other arm to support him or her from underneath B . Slowly straighten into a standing position C , keeping your abdominal stabilizers contracted throughout.

Carrying your child in this manner is acceptable for short periods, for example, if you want to take the child indoors or to bed. However, carrying children for extended

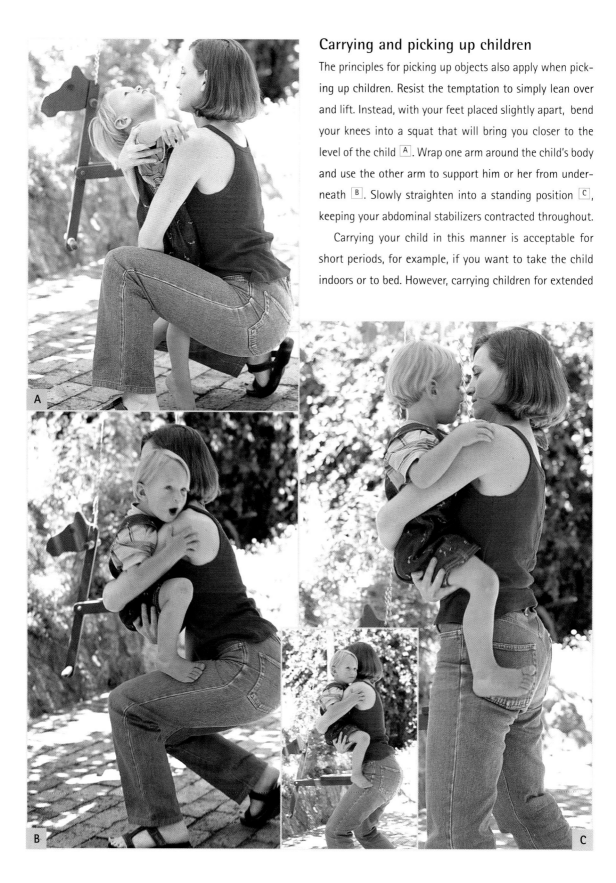

A

B

C

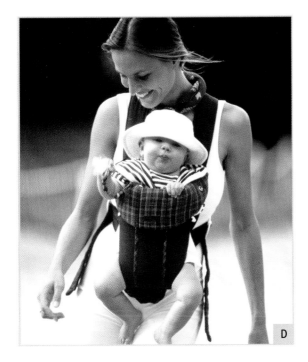

D

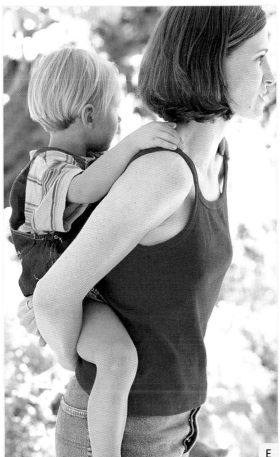

E

periods of time can pose a problem. While your baby is small you can carry your child in a papoose that distributes the weight evenly across the front of your body D. Make sure that you contract your abdominal stabilizers to support your lower back and that you don't hollow your back while carrying the baby. To this end, a papoose that has a wide band around your waist and puts most of the weight onto your hips is better than one with thin straps hanging from your shoulders.

It is better to carry an older child on your back for a length of time than on your hip E. If you carry a child on your hip, your spine will be pulled to one side putting undue pressure on surrounding structures. You should contract your abdominal stabilizers to protect your back, take breaks and alternate sides regularly.

During your breaks, move your back in the opposite direction to relieve some of the strain.

Walking

Aside from the obvious health benefits, walking allows you to keep your lower back in the neutral position without putting too much impact on the lower back. It also helps with neural mobility. Nerves may become impinged by structures around them; by keeping them mobile this is less likely to happen. Regular walks, approximately four times a week and lasting between 45–60 minutes at a time, will be of great benefit to you.

Walking offers a number of benefits, including:
- strengthening of muscles
- strengthening back muscles and mobilizing nerves
- keeping the cardiovascular system fit
- increasing bone density to minimize osteoporosis
- prevention of heart disease
- relief from stress
- lowering of cholesterol

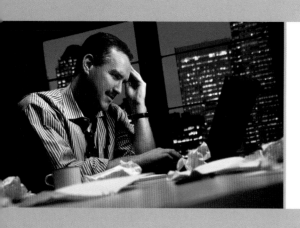

Diagnosis and Prevention

There are a number of lower back conditions that are considered relatively common problems. Should you frequently experience pain or discomfort in your lower back, the following case studies and explanations may help you identify your problem and determine how to prevent further injury. In extreme cases, it is recommended that you seek assistance from your doctor.

DISC PROLAPSE (SLIPPED DISC)

Causes: The intervertebral discs are most likely to be injured when the back is in the forward bending position and rotated at the same time. Repetitive or heavy lifting is also known to cause disc problems; less commonly, a fall or an injury.

Forward bending pushes the gel-like nucleus pulposus back, putting strain on the outer layer of the annulus fibrosus. Sustained bad posture in sitting can contribute to this condition. Truck drivers,

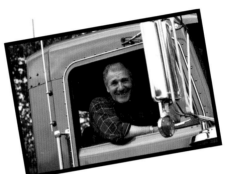

DISC PROLAPSE (SLIPPED DISC)

CASE STUDY 1

Mr Brown has never had a back problem before. Having recently experienced pain he describes his current problem as follows: "I just bent forward to pick up my cup of tea and I couldn't straighten up again. Two weeks ago I could still help lift a car out of a ditch next to the road. The pain is in my lower back. It is worse when I sit, and I really struggle to get up from the sitting position. It's slightly better when I've walked around a bit. Picking something up from the floor is impossible, it's very painful, but the pain is localized, I only feel it in my back."

sitting in a vibrating seat for long periods at a time, are likely to develop disc problems. Interestingly, coughing or sneezing can sometimes make you aware of a disc problem.

Symptoms: A constant, dull pain in the lower back, usually localized on one side. Sitting aggravates the pain, but this is sometimes only evident once you have stood up. Bending forwards increases the pain and is usually too painful to do. Pain is often worse in the morning, improving during the day. It may be difficult to stand up straight; you may find yourself leaning to one side, favoring the one that does not present pain.

Anatomy: The outer layer (annulus fibrosus) of the disc tears, usually at the back, and slightly to one side. As a result, the gel-like inner core (nucleus pulposus) pushes through (prolapse), putting pressure on the outermost layer of the disc causing it to bulge (see fig 1) and, in extreme cases, tear. This may exert pressure on structures lying close to the protruding disc, such as ligaments and the protective sheath covering the spinal nerve, leading

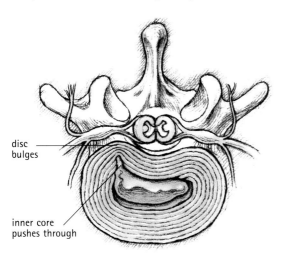

disc bulges

inner core pushes through

FIG 1   DISC PROLAPSE

to localized inflammation and swelling. Interestingly, the nucleus and layers of the disc do not have nerve endings and are therefore immune to pain. Only the outermost layer of the disc and structures around it register pain. As a result, it is very easy to injure the disc without feeling it; associated pain only becomes evident once the injury reaches the outermost layer of the disc. This explains why patients often say they cannot recall when they actually hurt their back.

Prevention: Once you have determined which activity caused your back problem, avoid it until your back is better. Carrying on with the same activity may cause further injury. If it is not possible to stop doing the activity, or you don't know what caused it, then it is very important that you do all activities correctly. If sitting caused it, then sit up straight, no slouching; if heavy lifting caused it, then make sure you bend your knees when lifting an object.

Short breaks between activities are vital. As disc problems are primarily brought about by forward movement, it is recommended that you take breaks and bend your back backwards to counteract and provide relief from forward bending.

When suffering from a slipped disc, it is preferable to walk and stand than to sit. Bed rest will help, but usually only in the first 24 hours.

When to consult a specialist: If you experience pain for longer than 24 hours, if you have "pins and needles" in your leg and/or if you experience acute pain in the mornings, consult a medical practitioner. Your doctor can prescribe a course of anti-inflammatory drugs that will help with the swelling and the pain.

Your doctor can also best determine whether it is in fact a back problem that you are experiencing, and refer you to the appropriate manual therapist. A manual therapist will identify your problem and treat your back to relieve pressure on the structures associated with the disc. He or she will also be able to give you advice on how to care for your back and how to prevent a recurrence of your specific condition.

DISC PROLAPSE WITH NERVE ROOT COMPRESSION

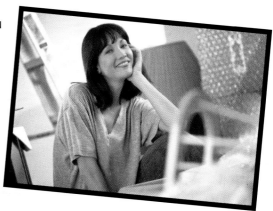

CASE STUDY 2

Mrs. Bell has experienced back pain before. "I get back pain every now and again, but nothing like this. The pain is usually just in my back and doesn't last for more than two days. If it is really painful, I'll go to the doctor and get a Voltaren (diclofenac) injection, which often helps. This time it's been longer than a week. The Voltaren injection didn't help at all. I think it's actually worse now than it was a week ago. I feel some pain in my back but the burning pain down my leg is unbearable. I also have a strange feeling in my foot, as if it is asleep. The pain in my leg sometimes wakes me up at night. Sitting and bending is very painful. After driving for a while, I struggle to get out of my car and move around. Standing is slightly more comfortable, but it is very difficult to do anything at all.

"It all started two weeks ago when we moved house. I was packing boxes and carrying them in and out of the house. I started to feel pain in my back and stopped picking up heavy boxes, but I had to carry on packing. Three days later the pain started in my leg. It feels like it's coming from my back, but I'm not sure."

DISC PROLAPSE
WITH NERVE ROOT COMPRESSION

Causes: The causes are similar to a normal disc prolapse, i.e. forward bending with rotation or heavy lifting. In this instance, the protrusion is more pronounced and presses on the nerve lying just outside the annulus. Disc prolapse with nerve root compression is a more serious injury and often occurs after several previous disc prolapse injuries.

Symptoms: In this instance the nerve pain is dominant and as a result symptoms may vary. A burning or numbing pain will be felt down one leg (radiating pain, see p30), and will be more obvious than any dull pain in the back. You are also likely to experience "pins and needles" in your foot. Your leg may feel weak, with a loss of feeling in certain areas. These symptoms are all a result of compression on the nerve.

Anatomy: As with the "simple" disc prolapse, the outer layer (annulus fibrosus) of the disc tears, allowing the gel-like inner core (nucleus pulposus) to push through. In this case, the protrusion is severe and it impinges on the spinal nerve (see fig 2) blocking the nerve's normal impulses to and from specific structures, such as the foot. Symptoms will vary according to the extent to which the disc has prolapsed, and where the nerve lies.

Prevention: Prevention for this condition is similar to the prevention for a simple disc prolapse. Avoid any activities that cause you pain and take short breaks to relieve strain on your back. If you've had previous disc problems, then you should start doing stretching and strengthening exercises to stabilize your back and prevent further injury.

When to consult a specialist: This injury is much more incapacitating than a "simple" disc prolapse and also takes longer to heal. If you experience prolonged pain, consult your doctor. He or she will be able to prescribe medication for pain relief and, if necessary, will refer you to a specialist for X-rays to confirm the diagnosis. If the condition is not too severe, you will be referred to a manual therapist qualified to treat your condition. Even after initial progress, conservative treatment with a manual therapist should continue.

If your symptoms are extreme (complete loss of sensation and weakness), you will be referred to a neurologist or a neurosurgeon. He or she may choose to operate to remove the disc protrusion, because if the nerve remains compressed for too long it could be damaged permanently. The procedure is called a laminectomy and by removing the protrusion impinging on the nerve, proper nerve function is restored and your symptoms improve.

Following an operation, it will be recommended that you consult a physiotherapist for rehabilitation and prevention of further injury.

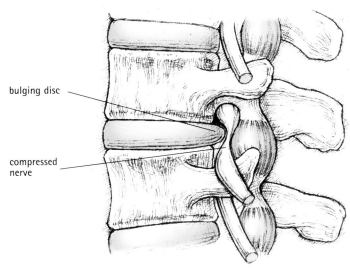

bulging disc

compressed nerve

FIG 2   DISC PROLAPSE WITH NERVE ROOT COMPRESSION

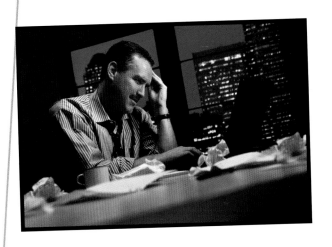

DEGENERATIVE DISC PROBLEMS

CASE STUDY 3

Mr Green has been working hard and has been under a lot of stress lately. He has the following complaint: "I've had back problems periodically for a long time. I've learned to live with it and I go to see someone if it gets too painful. It's always the same, the dull, stiff ache is in my back. In extreme cases it spreads right across my back and sometimes into my buttocks. I sometimes get a strange feeling down the back of my left leg. The leg pain is not half as bad as my back pain. Sitting for long periods always makes it difficult to get up and move again. When I'm on the move it's better, but if I do too much it becomes really painful. I've been fine lately, but yesterday I tripped over a loose brick in my driveway and my back has been incredibly sore since then."

DEGENERATIVE DISC PROBLEMS

Causes: As a natural phenomenon of the aging process, discs lose their water content and degenerate. As a result, tears occur in the outer lining of the disc (annulus fibrosus). Although these degenerative processes are part of the natural aging of the spine, some individuals' discs degenerate much faster than others. A genetic predisposition to having bad discs can be a risk factor for degenerative disc problems. However, activities that place physical pressure on the back, such as repetitive heavy lifting or movements executed incorrectly, are also contributing factors.

Symptoms: The primary symptom of a degenerative disc problem is midline back pain. Individuals may often experience radiated pain in the buttocks and/or pelvis. Pain is greater when sitting and standing than when lying down, which decreases the pressure on the degenerating disc. You may have difficulty finding a comfortable position when sitting or standing, and feel the need to constantly change positions. Bending and lifting, especially heavy items, aggravates the pain and rising from a chair may be problematic. An injury, such as jumping onto your feet from a height, or an abrupt move can present sudden, unexpected pain that would bring to light a degenerating disc problem.

Anatomy: The outer layer of the disc has thinned and become less elastic. The gel-like nucleus has lost some of its water content and is less pliable as a result (see figs 3 and 4). The cushioning function of the disc is ineffective and it does not absorb and distribute weight as before.

Prevention: Correcting your posture, incorporating mobility and stability exercises into your daily routine and making sure your stabilizers are activated correctly before and during any activity — all these things will reduce pressure on the disc.

When to consult a specialist: If you experience recurring problems with your back, you need only consult a medical practitioner when your symptoms change or if your pain does not ease. A doctor will be able to prescribe anti-inflammatory medication to help with the pain and swelling. He or she will also refer you to the appropriate manual therapist. A physiotherapist, for example, is qualified to advise you on the prevention of further injury. He or she can help with pain relief by helping you strengthen your stabilizers (easing some of the pressure on the disc) and developing an exercise program that will keep your vertebral column mobile.

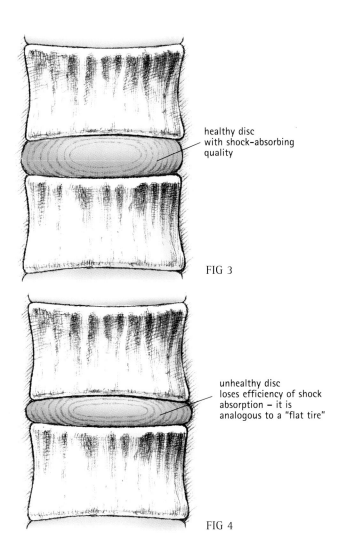

healthy disc with shock-absorbing quality

FIG 3

unhealthy disc loses efficiency of shock absorption – it is analogous to a "flat tire"

FIG 4

FACET JOINT SPRAIN OR SPONDYLOSIS

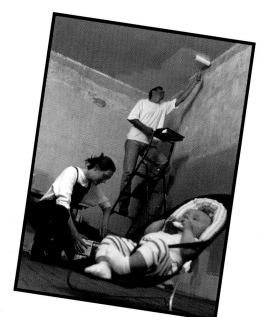

case study: 4

Mr Ross took a day off from work to do all the things that were long overdue at home. The next day he complained: "This morning when I woke up I couldn't move. If I lie still I don't feel anything, but turning in bed is extremely difficult and painful. Getting out of bed was difficult but after I had a shower, I seemed to have loosened up a bit. Sitting is actually quite pleasant, it feels less painful than standing, which is extremely uncomfortable. Yesterday I spent the last few hours of my day painting the ceiling, standing on a ladder looking up. I did feel slightly stiff in my back when I finished, but I went to bed early and only this morning was it really painful."

FACET JOINT SPRAIN AND SPONDYLOSIS

Causes: Facet joint sprain is caused by any activity that puts strain on the facet joints. Prolonged fully bent positions will overstretch the capsule and ligaments of the joint. An extreme hollow-back posture or extended periods of backward bending subject the facet joints to permanent compression, causing friction on the joint surfaces which, in turn, can lead to degeneration in the joints. Sports that have an excessive range of movement, such as ballet, gymnastics and golf, may result in facet joint problems. With age, these joints degenerate, making them more prone to injury and spondylosis.

Symptoms: Pain is usually localized over the area of the joint, but it can radiate up or down from there. You may experience muscle spasms in your back secondary to the joint sprain, which could give you symptoms, such as stiffness, and also radiate pain to other areas. Sitting brings relief. Standing and walking are not as comfortable. Lying down is comfortable, but turning in bed is difficult.

Anatomy: There are two different anatomical aspects of facet joint sprain. Side-flexion, rotation and/or extension carried out too quickly or held for long periods of time increase the compression load on the joint, damaging the cartilage. On the other hand, sustained side-flexion and rotation, sometimes even flexion, puts excessive strain on the ligaments and capsule around the joint, eventually causing them to tear (see fig 5). In this case, the damage done to the ligaments is similar to what occurs with an acute traumatic event, such as an ankle sprain.

Prevention: If you experience any of the aforementioned symptoms, stay away from the activities that cause pain, such as standing and bending backwards. You'll find relief with the rounding of your back, e.g. lying down and pulling your knees towards your chest. Basic preventative guidelines include correcting your posture, especially extreme lordosis-kyphosis and sway-back posture. Do not spend hours in a backward-bending position. Take short breaks, and bend your back in the opposite direction during these breaks to relieve strain.

When to consult a specialist: It would be wise to consult a medical practitioner if you experience prolonged pain over a number of days. If you are struggling to sleep or finding it difficult to function during the day, you may need to take anti-inflammatory medication. If the joint has experienced degenerative changes, they will be evident on an X-ray. This will not necessarily alter your treatment, but it will confirm the diagnosis and you will be referred to a qualified manual therapist.

A manual therapist will work with you to loosen tight ligament capsules. Through manipulation he or she will be able to increase the circulation around your joints, easing some of the swelling, decreasing stiffness and providing relief from pain. He or she will further help you to correct your posture and help train your muscles to support your lower back.

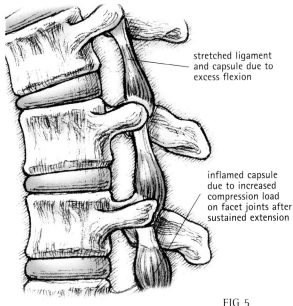

stretched ligament and capsule due to excess flexion

inflamed capsule due to increased compression load on facet joints after sustained extension

FIG 5

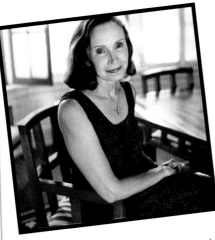

case study 6

Mrs. Gordon was diagnosed with instability of her lower back four years ago. She explains her back problem as follows: "I'm used to my back being uncomfortable. I've learned to live with it. some days I barely feel it and other days I can't move. I try to do things correctly and have even learned to avoid some movements altogether, but sometimes I forget and end up doing things I shouldn't. This is when my back gets painful again. The pain is restricted largely to my lower back, and seems more intense on the left. Other times it can be more evident on the right. sometimes I get a sharp pain down my leg but it comes and goes. I don't have any leg pain now as I'm standing here. However, all my movements are painful: sitting for long periods, standing for long periods, even walking for a long period of time is extremely painful. If I lie down, I experience some relief but I find it difficult to move if I've been still for too long. I have a heat pack and using it helps for a while, but it doesn't take the pain away."

INSTABILITY OF THE LOWER BACK (SPONDYLOLISTHESIS)

Causes: Spondylolisthesis can present either as a result of a congenital anomaly or, in some cases, as the result of a stress fracture suffered during childhood. Essentially, a defect in the pars interarticularis leads, in extreme cases, to a displacement of the vertebral bodies, which can compromise the spinal cord. Children involved in certain sports that put a lot of stress on the back, such as gymnastics, weight-lifting and football, have been known to suffer a higher incidence of spondylolysis, the precursor to spondylolisthesis. Dysfunctional discs and compromised joints may also lead to a degenerative condition in the adult.

Symptoms: In some cases, this condition can be completely asymptomatic. If symptoms do present, you may find activities such as walking up stairs or down an incline painful. Any movement effected for a long period of time may also cause pain. You may experience attacks of severe pain with symptom-free periods in between.

Anatomy: Spondylolisthesis most commonly occurs in the segment of the lumbar spine known as L5 which lies above the first sacral segment, or S1 (see p22). The term means "forward shift of the spine" and refers to the displacement of the vertebral bodies resulting from the loss of bony continuity between the superior and inferior facets (spondylolysis). In extreme cases, the pars interarticularis is compromised on both sides of the vertebra and the capsule and ligaments are not strong enough to prevent the forward glide of the vertebra (spondylolisthesis). As a result the top vertebra glides further forward on the bottom one, putting immense strain on the disc, which is now the only major structure preventing the vertebrae from gliding off each other and compromising the spinal cord.

Unstable joints don't respond well to movement.

Prevention: If you have already been diagnosed with spondylolisthesis, it is very difficult to prevent symptoms completely. A back brace might help to limit movement, but in the long run it will weaken your stabilizing muscles. If you have this instability, it is important that you alter your lifestyle and do things in moderation, correct your posture and prevent excessive range of movement wherever possible. Less stress at the L5 level will result in fewer symptoms.

To treat the problem you need a program of muscle-stabilizing exercises. Your own strengthened stabilizing muscles will support your lower back far better than a lumbar brace would.

When to consult a specialist: A medical practitioner will be able to diagnose your condition, request X-rays and prescribe pain medication, but to help you strengthen your back and limit excess movement you need to consult a qualified manual therapist, who will monitor your instability and devise an exercise program.

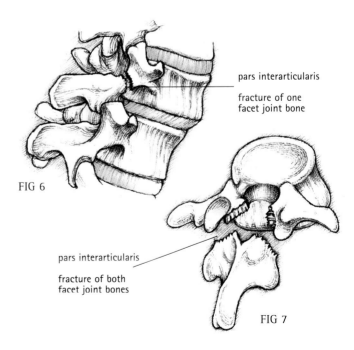

pars interarticularis

fracture of one facet joint bone

FIG 6

pars interarticularis

fracture of both facet joint bones

FIG 7

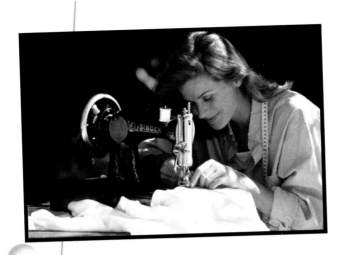

PROBLEMS AFTER A BACK OPERATION

case study 7

Six months ago Mrs. Kennedy had an operation (laminectomy) due to pain in her lower back stemming from severe nerve root compression. She explains her problem as follows: "It feels like just before the operation, but not as bad. I have a pain that goes down my leg that feels kind of tight, like a pulled muscle. It is definitely worse when I haven't moved for a while, and in the morning it takes me some time before I can move properly. Getting up and doing things does help but certain movements, such as driving and keeping my foot on the accelerator, are very uncomfortable. My leg feels numb but I do not have the 'pins and needles' sensation in my foot that I experienced before the operation."

PROBLEMS AFTER A BACK OPERATION

Causes: A common cause of symptoms following a back operation is the stiffening of muscles and ligaments in the back due to lack of movement. It could be that they have developed scar tissue (fibrosis) as a result of the laminectomy, impairing smooth movement and causing a "pull" or strain in a specific area. Common structures affected by scar tissue are the spinal nerves and their pathways.

However, it is very difficult to establish the true cause of back pain following an operation and a full medical evaluation is recommended.

Symptoms: The symptoms will differ according to the type of injury. With the stiffening up of structures, the back will commonly register pain in the morning, before loosening up during the day. Symptoms could manifest themselves as radiating pain down the leg or localized back pain. There will invariably be a tight, pulling feeling at the end of back movements, as structures tighten up. You may also experience the same symptoms down your leg that you had before your operation.

Anatomy: Scar tissue is a normal process of healing, and is to be expected after a back operation. However, due to forced bed rest and lack of movement, scar tissue can often detrimentally affect important structures such as muscles and nerves. In many cases after a laminectomy, the spinal nerve thickens due to fibrosis and is no longer able to glide smoothly in and out of the small intervertebral foramen (see fig 8). This causes local pain at the point of tension or radiated pain down the leg along which the nerve extends.

Prevention: Keep fit! And make sure you always do things correctly. Do not remain in one position for long periods of time without stretching your back in the opposite direction to relieve strain. Take breaks regularly. Make sure you are using your transverse abdominal muscles correctly throughout the day. Your back will be more prone to injury after an operation, so look after it. A back operation should always be a last resort, but if it comes to this, proper rehabilitation is essential.

When to consult a specialist:

If you have had an operation and you experience another injury, consult a medical practitioner. He or she will diagnose the problem and refer you to the appropriate manual therapist. A manual therapist will help with the loosening up of structures and will work out an exercise program to maintain mobility. Treatment will be directed at the relief of pain, correcting the faulty structure, and finally, preventing the same injury from recurring. If your symptoms are not severe but persistent, you may need an exercise program to strengthen your stabilizers.

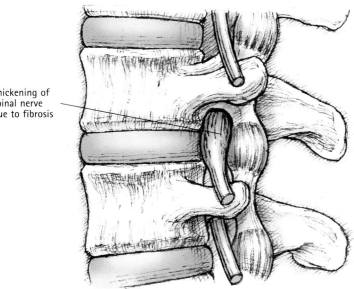

Thickening of spinal nerve due to fibrosis

FIG 8

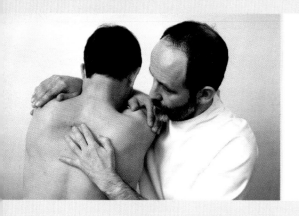

Therapies and Practitioners

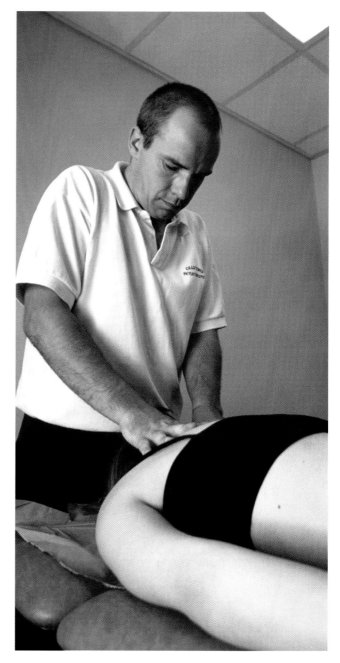

There are numerous practitioners and therapists who claim to have a solution for back problems. Some rely on more orthodox Western medicine, while others draw on the alternative treatments that stem from Eastern cultures. This chapter contains a brief outline of several of these disciplines, focusing primarily on those that contain a physical component, and will give you an idea of what the treatments involve and how they might prevent back pain.

PHYSIOTHERAPY

Physiotherapy is a branch of medical treatment that is anchored in movement sciences and concerned with the function of multiple body systems. Physiotherapists evaluate musculoskeletal problems and the impact of injury, disease or disorders on movement and function. They employ physical methods to encourage healing and restoration of movement, and often work in close collaboration with a medical doctor.

A physiotherapist will be able to assess your imbalances and potential problems, and devise exercise programs targeting your individual back complaints. He or she may use techniques to manipulate the soft tissue (muscles and ligaments), joints, fascia and nerves, as well as exercise methods to improve your movement and posture. Physiotherapists adopt state-of-the-art diagnostic and assessment procedures and tools to plan preventative and therapeutic courses of intervention. However, they do not only treat a specific problem; they encourage patients to assume responsibility for their health and participate in problem-solving and treatment.

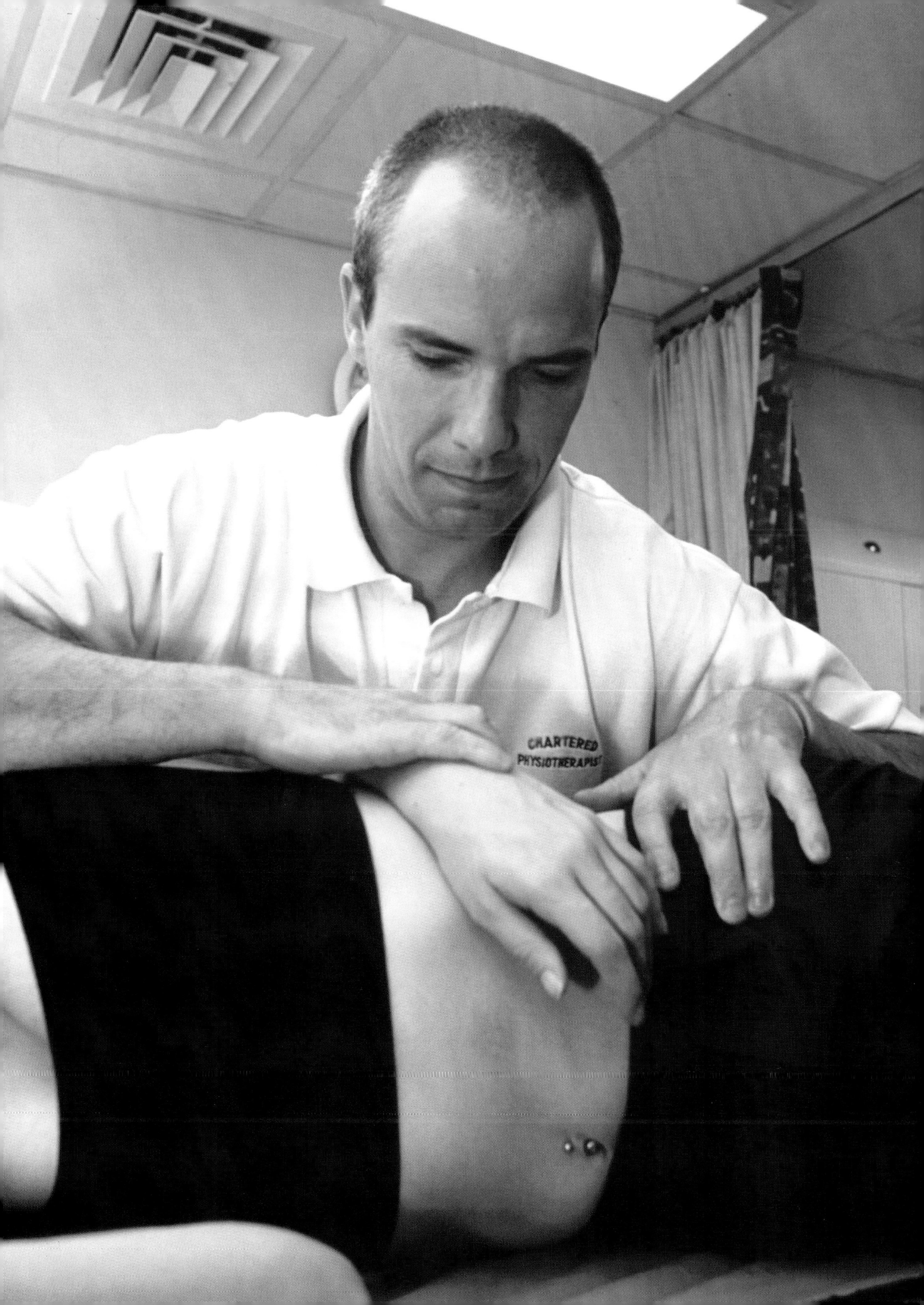
CHARTERED
PHYSIOTHERAPIST

CHIROPRACTIC

Chiropractic is a branch of the healing arts that is concerned with human health and the prevention of disease. Chiropractors consider a person as an integrated being, but give special attention to spinal biomechanics, musculoskeletal, neurological, vascular and nutritional relationships. Primarily, they focus on problems or diseases associated with the neuro-musculoskeletal system, therefore commonly treated conditions include strains/sprains, headaches, disc problems, sciatica and arthritis, among others.

One of the chiropractor's primary tools is the chiropractic adjustment. Through spinal manipulation, the chiropractor can gently and skilfully direct a specific force to restore normal range of motion to a joint that is being restricted by muscles or fibrous adhesions. Abnormal nerve signals caused by the restriction, which creates interference with normal function, can then be eliminated. Once regular motion is restored, other systems and structures that have compensated for the problem can return to normal.

Studies have shown that the manual techniques can trigger the release of natural painkillers known as endorphins, and that swelling, inflammation and pain can reduce significantly after an adjustive intervention. The effects of a chiropractic adjustment may be felt long distances from the point at which it was delivered, e.g. the elimination

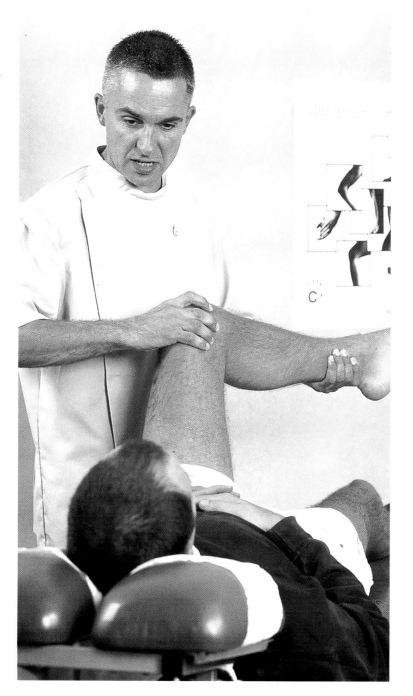

of a chronic headache after an adjustment of the vertebrae in the lower back. Because a chiropractor's approach is conservative and designed to be as non-invasive as possible, it may take several adjustments over a period of time to restore balance to a specific area.

OSTEOPATHY

During the mid-late19th century, an American doctor, Andrew Taylor Still, discovered the principles on which osteopathy is based. It was Dr. Still himself who in 1874 assigned the symbolic label "Osteopathy" to his discoveries. Osteopathy is an alternative medicine based primarily on the manual diagnosis and treatment of impaired function resulting from a loss of movement in the musculoskeletal structures. It aims to restore function to the organism by treating the cause of pain and imbalance. To achieve this goal the osteopath relies on palpation, massage and manipulation techniques, and works with the position and mobility of the structures. An osteopath may develop an exercise program to improve your posture and every treatment includes education on the prevention of problems.

Another (and more controversial) method of treatment that has developed from traditional osteopathy is Cranial Osteopathy, also known as Craniosacral Therapy or CST. CST focuses on the nervous system, especially the membranes and the fluid — called cerebrospinal fluid or CSF — that surrounds the brain and the spinal cord. CSF moves in a smooth, rhythmic motion, and as it moves, expanding and contracting movements occur in other parts of the body. A normal rhythm is associated with the body's own healing system, and is affected by the heart and respiratory rate.

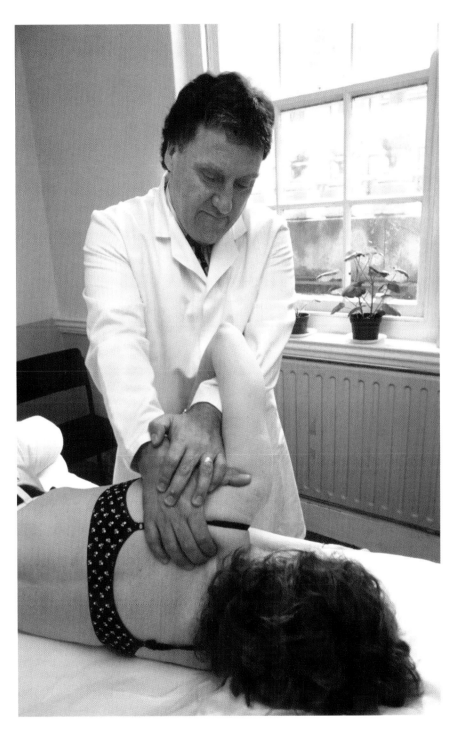

Therapists claim to be able to feel abnormalities or blockages in the movements and use gentle pressure on the bones of the head, spine, chest, ribcage, arms and legs to alter the impulses and restore a normal rhythm.

ROLFING AND
STRUCTURAL INTEGRATION

Structural Integration, also known as Rolfing, was first developed by American biochemist, Dr. Ida Rolf, some 50 years ago. It is an alternative therapy based on deep tissue manipulation and movement education, with the intention of re-aligning the human body within the field of gravity.

Rolfing is not a cure for any particular disease or physical problem, but is rather a systematic approach that attempts to restore balance to the entire body. This approach works on the premise that the body's connective tissue (fascia) forms a continuous web throughout the body and can be manipulated and actually reshaped. Dr. Rolf argued that reshaping was necessary because the body, over time, was pulled out of alignment by the effects of gravity. When this occurs, it is the muscles rather than the bones that bear the weight of gravity. The body's fascia loses some of its pliability and becomes thickened and hardened; eventually they act more like binding straps and the muscles atrophy, or shrink.

Treatment usually consists of 10 weekly sessions, each lasting 60–90 minutes. During treatments, the practitioner applies pressure with fingertips, hands, knuckles and elbows and reworks the fascial tissue of the patient's entire body until it becomes elastic and pliable again. This loosening of the adhesions in the fascia allows the muscles to lengthen and return to their normal, vertical alignment. It also restores a greater freedom of movement.

The benefits of Rolfing can include pain relief, greater range of motion, increased breathing capacity and improved body definition. Although practitioners do not attempt to cure specific complaints, many people claim that relief is obtained from chronic back conditions as well as neck, shoulder and joint pain.

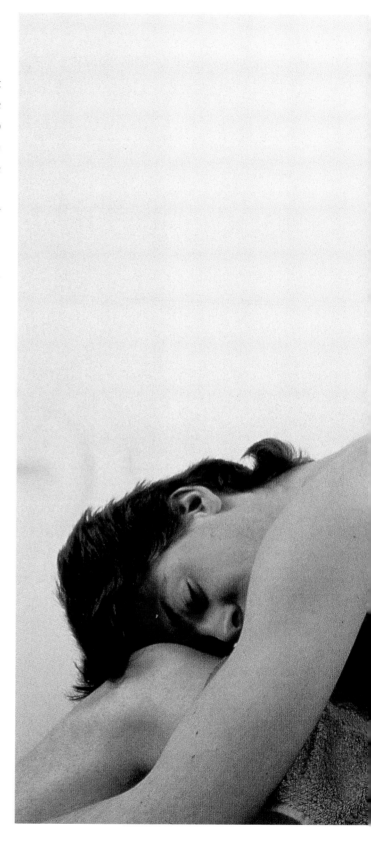

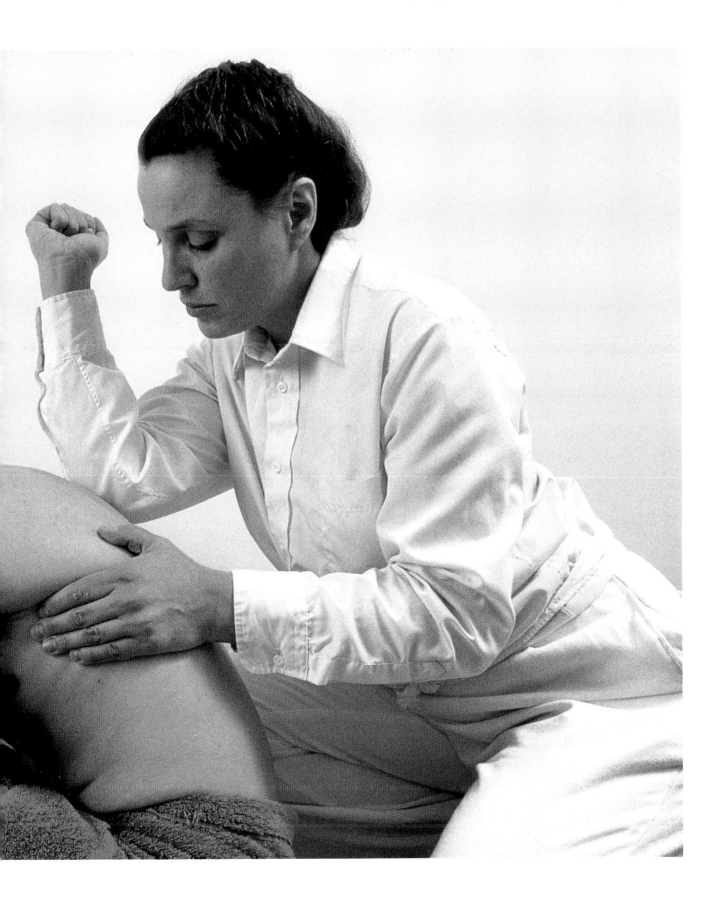

HELLERWORK

Hellerwork is named after its founder, Joseph Heller, an engineer and former disciple of Rolfing. In the 1970s, Heller left the practice of Rolfing to develop his own variation of deep tissue massage therapy. He believed that manipulation alone was insufficient and felt that it did not provide long-term or lasting results. Heller designed a structured, thematic approach consisting of 11 sessions that focused on both the body and the mind. He incorporated educational aspects to treatment, providing guidance on how to move properly, and encouraged his patients to examine the important role that habits and emotions play in our health.

Like Rolfing, Hellerwork uses manipulation to restore the body's original balance. During the first three sessions the practitioner applies pressure with his or her hands, finger, and sometimes even elbows, working on the chest area to promote more natural breathing. The practitioner will also engage the patient in a discussion of how certain emotional states can affect breathing.

The next four sessions form what are essentially regarded as the core sessions. They involve the manipulation and loosening of the muscles in the legs, pelvis, spine, neck and head. The final four sessions, referred to as the integrative sessions, work towards integrating the physical realignments achieved through manipulation with the client's own

awareness of emotional and situational problems that can impact on the physical body. By the end of the program, patients will not only have been instructed on how to sit, stand and walk, they will also have an awareness of the importance of proper movement.

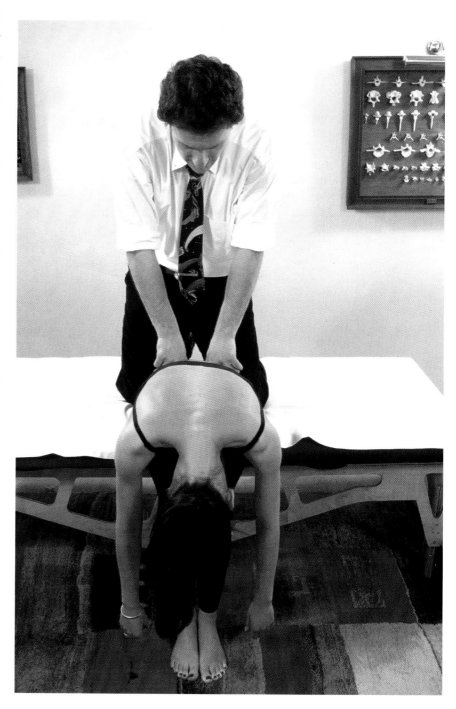

FELDENKRAIS METHOD

Feldenkrais is a form of body awareness and control that can benefit those suffering from neurological and musculoskeletal problems. It is also a useful means of decreasing stress and increasing self-awareness, self-esteem and general well-being.

Feldenkrais is a preventive therapy, not a treatment, based upon an obvious concept that many of us ignore. The body tends to fall into habitual ways of doing things, from sitting at a computer to picking up a child to standing at the kitchen counter chopping an onion. While these types of movement are effective, they generally call for more range of movement and strain than absolutely necessary. We often don't realize that we are unnecessarily tensing up certain parts of our body or that, in an effort to protect an injured area, we are putting undue stress on other areas.

In Feldenkrais classes, students are made aware of the way in which they stand, reach, turn, or bend. They are informed about other options that make everyday movements more conservative and effective without repercussions in other areas of the body. The aim of the course is to enhance awareness so that the principles can be applied in everyday movement.

ALEXANDER TECHNIQUE

Developed in 1904 by Australian actor Frederick Matthias Alexander, the Alexander Technique is a specific method of adjusting and correcting habitual misaligned body posture in order to relieve muscle tension and allow the body to move with greater ease and efficiency.

Having noticed that his breathing and voice were adversely affected by the tense way in which he held himself on stage, Alexander developed a straightforward system of balancing his head, neck and back which not only improved his performance but contributed to his overall general health. His technique is based on the principle that the mind and body function as a whole. According to Alexander, the habits of bad posture that everyone falls into as they age can result in many of the everyday aches and pains that we experience. This is attributed to the imbalances created by the incorrect positioning of the head in relation to the neck and torso which, in turn, results in inefficient or misplaced muscular effort and unnecessary muscular tension.

Practitioners, referred to as teachers, work to undo these ingrained bad habits and replace them with the correct, natural movements of early childhood. They rely on a process of re-education imparted during one-on-one sessions held several times a week. The way in which a student uses his or her body is studied and the teacher provides an awareness of muscular tension, posture and correct forms of movement. The aim is for this improved movement to become second nature. The technique is particularly popular with performers, such as actors, dancers and singers, who wish to improve their performance and avoid injury.

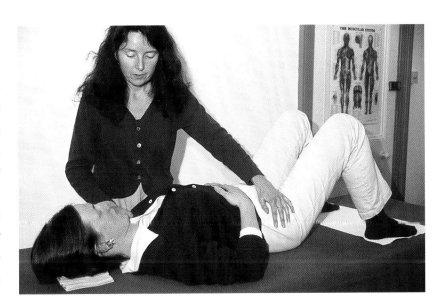

YOGA

The word "yoga" is derived from the Sanskrit language and means "to unite" or "to harmonize". Yoga is a psychological, physiological and spiritual discipline that has been an integral part of Indian culture for thousands of years. The ancient Yogis developed the system as a means of achieving harmony within themselves and in relation to their environment. They believed that by working with the body and breath, control over the mind, emotions and general well-being could be achieved.

In essence, yoga is a philosophy as well as a methodology of life. It is also a system of health maintenance that is long-lasting and cultivates a sense of happiness and fulfilment. It achieves this by teaching individuals how to tap into inner energy reserves and generate health and happiness from within. Yoga enhances health and youthfulness of the body, and clarity of the mind. As a result, regular practice can help counter the physical effects of aging, ease aggravated stress or tension and improve posture, movement and balance.

The different postures in yoga are together designed to benefit every anatomical structure, system and organ in the body. Flexibility exercises are helpful in preventing and/or alleviating muscular tension, while the use of controlled, deep breathing helps to counter any irregularity of breathing associated with stress. Yoga provides a comprehensive system of exercise that stretches, strengthens, tones, helps to align and improves the health of the entire body. It also develops a state of mental calmness and emotional stability. According to yoga philosophy, health is first an inner state. This means that health of the nerves, glands and vital organs determines how healthy a person looks and feels. Yoga is non-competitive and allows each person to work within personal limits.

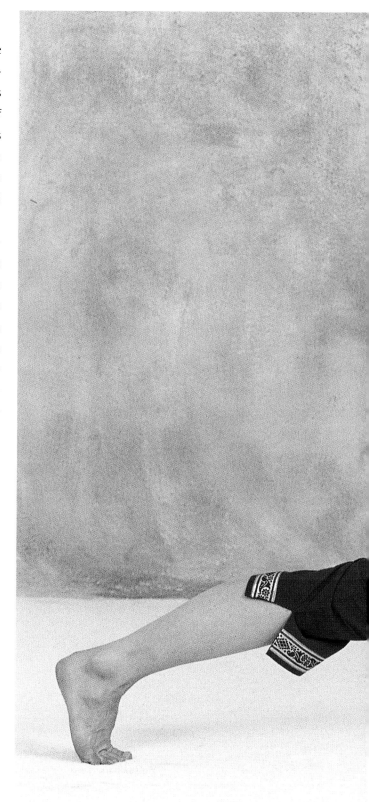

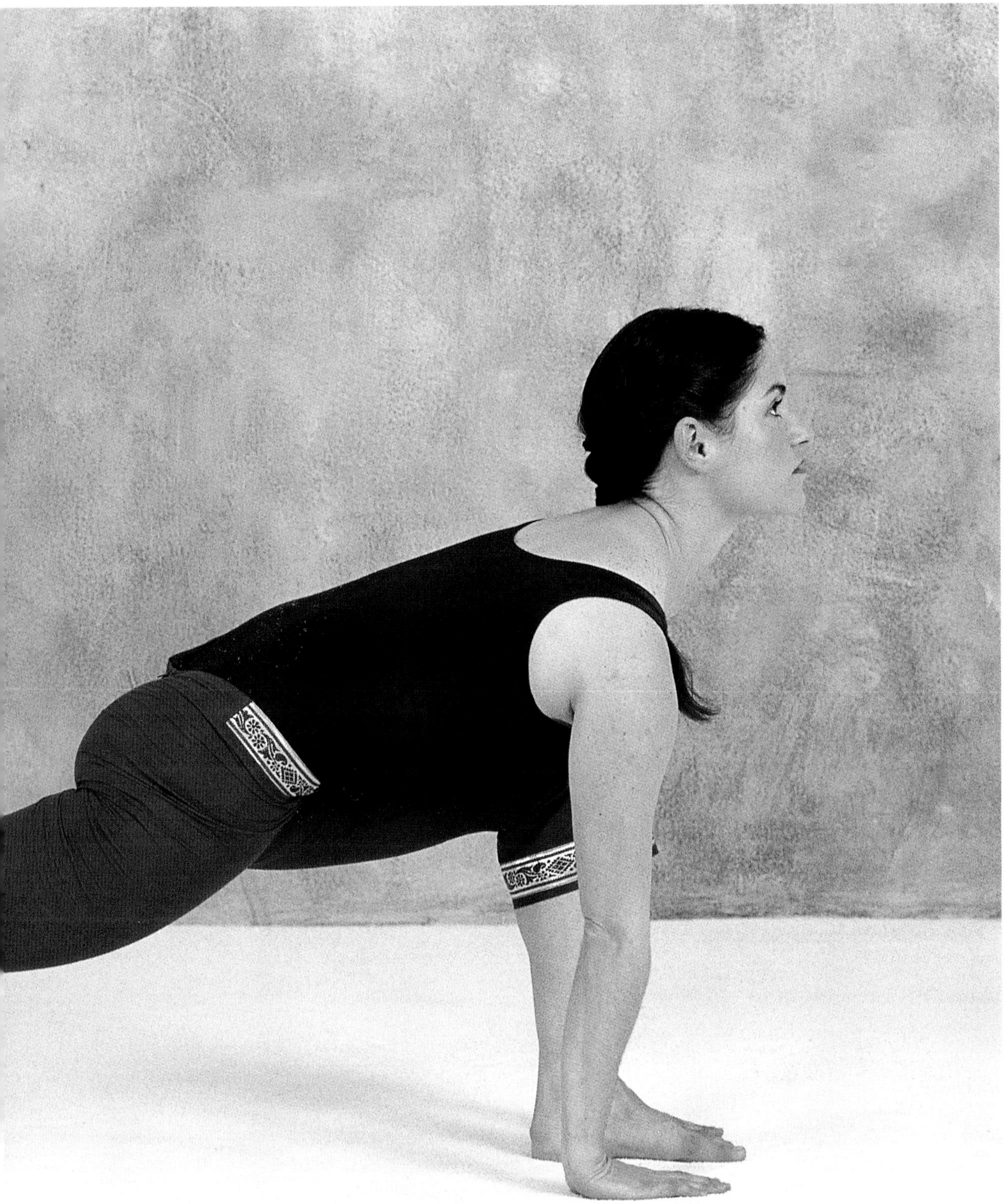

PILATES

Joseph Pilates, the founder of Pilates, was born in Germany in 1880. He was a frail child, who suffered from rickets, asthma and rheumatic fever. Determined to become stronger, he dedicated himself to building both body and mind through practices which included yoga, zen and ancient Greek and Roman exercises. His conditioning regime worked and he became an accomplished gymnast, skier, boxer and diver.

Stationed in England during World War I, Pilates became a nurse. During this time, he designed a unique system of hooking springs and straps to a hospital bed in order to help his disabled and immobilized patients regain strength and movement. It was through these experiments that he recognized the importance of training the core abdominal and back muscles to stabilize the torso and allow the entire body to move freely. This experimentation provided the foundation for his style of conditioning as well as the specialized exercise equipment associated with the Pilates method.

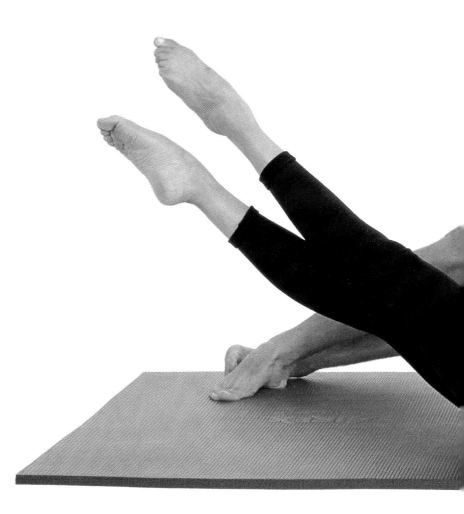

Pilates is a form of strength and flexibility training that can be carried out by individuals at any level of fitness. It promotes a feeling of physical and mental well-being and also develops inner physical awareness. It helps to prevent and treat injuries, improve posture, and increase flexibility, circulation and balance.

A treatment can range anywhere from 10 to 30 sessions. During the initial meeting, an instructor will analyze the client's posture and movement and design a specific training program. There are over 500 exercises that were developed by Joseph Pilates, many of which include concentration, centering, flowing movement and breath. Two primary exercise machines are used for

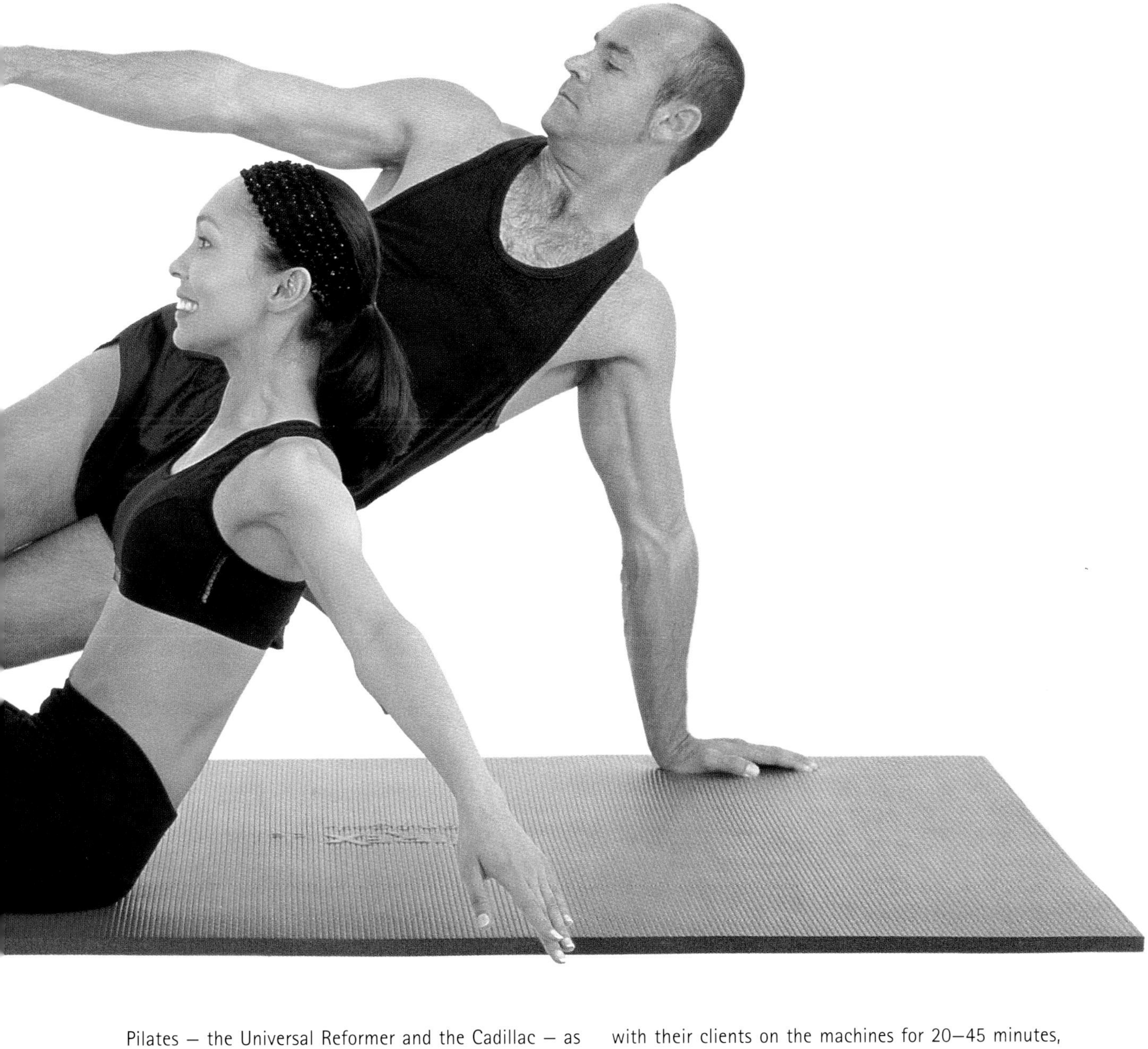

Pilates – the Universal Reformer and the Cadillac – as well as several other smaller pieces of equipment. The Reformer resembles a single bed frame and is equipped with a carriage that slides back and forth, and adjustable springs that are used to regulate tension and resistance. Cables, bars, straps and pulleys allow the exercises to be done from a variety of positions. Instructors usually work with their clients on the machines for 20–45 minutes, during which time they observe and provide feedback about alignment, breathing and precision of movement.

Once the basics are learned from an instructor, it is possible to train at home using videos. Exercise equipment for home use is also available and many exercises can be carried out on a mat.

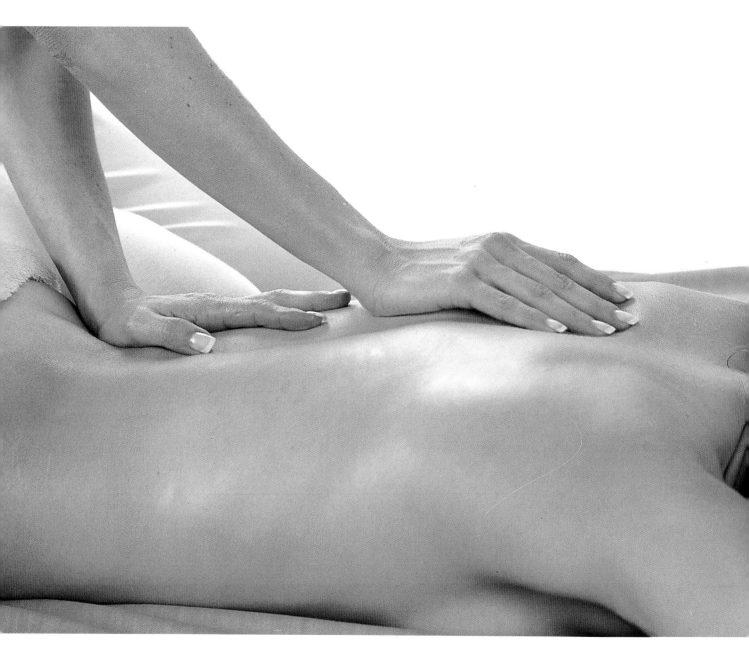

SWEDISH MASSAGE

Although therapeutic massage can be traced back 5000 years to the ancient cultures of Egypt, Greece and Rome, Swedish massage, widely used in the West today, was popularized by Per Hendrik Ling in the early 19th century. In 1813, Ling founded the Central Institute of Gymnastics in Stockholm. He used his understanding of gymnastics, anatomy and physiology together with the knowledge available from the Chinese, Greek and Egyptian systems to develop a modern, formalized method of massage.

Massage is a form of touch therapy that involves manipulation (physical movement) of the soft tissues of the body, such as the skin, tendons, ligaments and muscles. Although one is inclined to think that the bones in the body are not affected by massage, this is untrue.

A tense muscle can place a bone or joint under pressure as it is "pulled" by the muscle. Ligaments that join the muscle to the bone are tighter than they should be and very little circulation can get to the bony structures because the capillaries and veins are contracted, much like a hose pipe when it is squeezed. The body needs all the oxygen it can get, and this is carried in the bloodstream through the veins, arteries and capillaries. When a stimulating massage takes place, the transportation of the necessary fluids is improved, either by removing toxins or by bringing fresh oxygenated blood to the body part that is being manipulated. Conversely, a gentle massage brings about relaxation and helps to reduce excessive emotional and physical stress, factors that are known to aggravate or increase the symptoms of back pain.

THAI MASSAGE

Thai massage is one of the ancient healing arts of traditional Thai medicine and has its roots in Indian Ayurvedic medicine and yoga. Traditional Thai massage fluidly blends gentle rocking, rhythmic acupressure and assisted stretches to relax and revitalize the body and mind.

The body's energy lines are the focus of Thai massage. Although similar to the meridians of Chinese acupressure, Thai energy lines, known as *sen*, are believed to flow through the entire body and are therefore not asso-

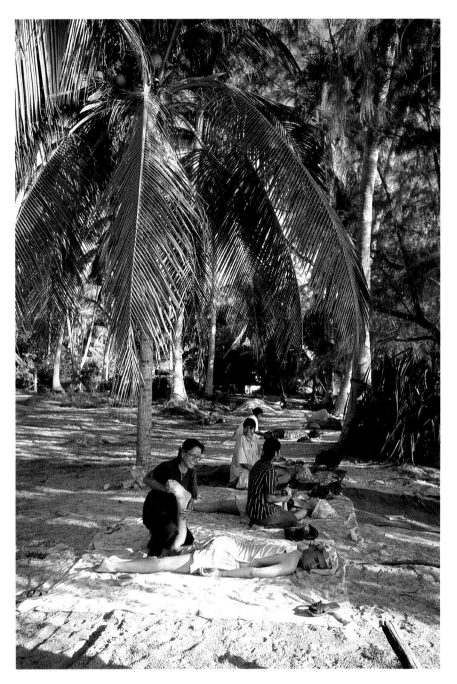

ciated with specific organs. The masseuse exerts pressure on the energy lines and pressure points along them, using the palms, thumbs, feet and occasionally elbows. Pressure therapy is combined with passive stretching movements that relax the body, releasing tension and increasing flexibility.

111

stress or weight being put through them; water aerobics can also be beneficial in this instance.

Neck pain can, however, be exacerbated by swimming if your head is held out of the water. This is often the case with swimmers who prefer breast stroke. It is important that you learn to swim with your face in the water – in this way keeping your cervical spine in line with the lumbar vertebrae – only lifting it for breath. Alternatively consider swimming backstroke or freestyle.

Cycling is another form of exercise that can aggravate neck pain as the head is held up to see where you are going. Lowering your seat or raising your handlebars can reduce the amount of strain you place on your neck during this activity. Remember that any position that is held for an extended period of time can cause muscle tension that may lead to pain and that constant movement or positional changes are necessary.

Q My husband is quite a fitful sleeper and has woken up on occasion with a very stiff neck, hardly able to turn his head. He refuses to go for treatment, but thankfully always recovers in a few days. Could this painful condition have anything to do with his sleeping pattern?

A This condition, known as acute wry neck syndrome, is quite common among both adults and children. Many people move around surprisingly vigorously during their sleep. It is possible in these cases that they twist their necks into an unnatural position putting strain on the cervical muscles and/or joints. On the other hand, during deep, dreaming sleep, the muscles relax to such an extent that the neck can fall into an awkward position, similarly causing strain. If the neck remains in this position for several hours, it is likely that one of the cervical facet joints could become slightly displaced. In this case the cartilage flap inside the joint is hooked on the opposite flap, preventing the joint from returning to the resting position. Physical treatment (massage, physiotherapy or heat applications) will most certainly speed up recovery, but in most cases the pain will subside in a matter of days (in some instances, up to 10 days or more). If the pain does not ease, or radiated pain is felt in the arms or hands, then it is advisable to seek advice from a medical practitioner or manual therapist.

Q I was involved in a minor car accident about six months ago and suffered a whiplash injury. I wore a neck brace for three weeks and my doctor assured me that I would be fine, but I still frequently experience neck pain. Why is this?

A Whiplash is an injury to the neck resulting from a sudden thrusting forward and snapping back of the unsupported head. Automobile accidents are the main contributor to whiplash incidents and the injury is most commonly sustained from a rear or side impact. What many people do not know is that the force of impact experienced by the driver or passenger is generally two and a half times greater than the impact on the vehicle. A common misconception is that if there is no vehicle damage, there would be equally little or no injury to those inside the car.

Studies indicate that rapid changes in the pressure of the spinal column cause damage to the nerves. In extreme cases the spine can be fractured or dislocated requiring surgery. In less severe impacts, victims can experience mild muscle strain but continue to suffer symptoms (headaches, low back pain, neck pain, nausea, dizziness, "pins and needles") for months after the accident. Pain medication may provide some relief, but in most cases it is recommended to seek treatment from a physiotherapist. The soft tissue damaged or torn in a whiplash injury can become stiff as a result of the healing process. A qualified therapist will use manual techniques to mobilize the stiff joints and muscles which are causing you pain and discomfort.

A good preventive measure is to ensure that the headrests in your car are at the correct height. A headrest should be at least as high as the head's center of gravity, i.e. just above the ears. A headrest that sits behind the neck can potentially cause more damage as it serves as a blunt force compounding the effects of whiplash.

Q Can depression be a contributing factor when it comes to backache?

A Psychological and physical illness are quite often linked and it is not uncommon for depression to manifest itself as physical pain, especially back pain. When you are tired, drained and/or depressed it seems to take too much effort to sit or stand upright and your posture increasingly deviates from the ideal norm. Sustained bad posture affects the alignment of the spine and can lead to back problems over and above psychosomatic back pain.

In instances of severe depression, direct treatment of an associated back complaint will not provide long-term relief. The individual concerned should consider seeking advice from a doctor or psychotherapist, possibly combined with a course of antidepressants.

On the other hand, back pain that persists over a long period of time can lead to depression and this will need treatment in its own right.

Q Do neck braces or collars and back braces help relieve back pain? How?

A Neck and back braces have their place and can relieve pain, but they can also be detrimental if worn for a long period of time. Neck braces are often used after motor vehicle accidents to support the neck and allow the healing of strained or torn soft tissue. The length of time they are worn depends on the extent of damage, but the period does not usually extend beyond a few weeks. Neck and back braces are also worn after spinal surgery and in this instance offer support to the spine until the patient has fully recovered. In any instance where a brace is required, it is essential that it be fitted by a qualified therapist or practitioner. Wearing a brace incorrectly can compound an existing problem and do more harm than good.

It is generally not recommended that you wear a back brace to relieve lower back pain. Although the brace will support the spine temporarily it will weaken the stabilizing muscles and leave you more vulnerable to injury and pain in the long run. Back pain is often associated with weakness in the stabilizing muscles of the back, particularly the transverse abdominus (see pp40–41).

Occasionally, back braces can provide some relief from back pain in manual workers. This is because it can act as a reminder not to hold a flexed position and not to twist when lifting. It is important in these cases, however, that the brace is only worn during heavy work and not for extended periods of time.

Q I have heard that my diet can have an influence on back pain. Is this true?

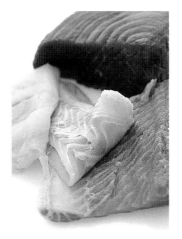
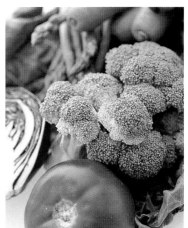
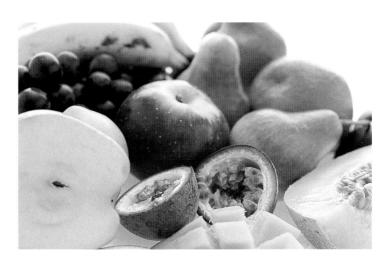

A Pain is often the result of inflammation, which is the body's response to injury. A healthy, balanced diet is essential for the health of all the body's structure (muscles, cartilage, bone, etc.) and any deficiencies can contribute to injury and degeneration. Diet can also affect our inflammatory response. Red meat and animal fats are believed to increase the inflammatory response, while oily fish such as sardines, mackerel, herring and salmon are particularly good for reducing inflammation.

It is generally recommended that you eat a diet rich in fruit, vegetables, garlic, onions and fish. You should avoid caffeine, processed foods and red meat. Fizzy drinks, coffee, chocolate and smoking are risk factors for reduced bone density. Vitamin and mineral supplements can help prevent deficiencies; in fact, glucosamine sulphate is one of the basic compounds in cartilage and has been shown to delay osteoarthritis.

There are also a number of patients who have found relief from arthritic pain by cutting out the foods in the nightshade family. While this does not help everyone it can be worth a try; it has dramatically improved some patients' symptoms. The foods in question are tomatoes, potatoes, eggplant and peppers, and they should be cut out for a month while symptoms are monitored.

Q My husband experiences regular back pain. Should he stop working until it goes away?

A In the past it was recommended that back pain sufferers go to bed, take painkillers and wait for the pain to subside. Unfortunately this was not good advice as tissues need movement for circulation, nutrition and drainage, and muscles need to be used or they become weak. It was found that people who did not stay in bed recovered more quickly. As a result of this finding, practitioners now frequently recommend that patients avoid long periods of rest as this can delay healing.

Your husband needs to listen to his body and do as much movement and exercise as feels comfortable. With acute, severe back pain it is a good idea for him to lie still on his back (if this is comfortable) with his knees bent for half an hour to an hour and then to slowly walk around a few minutes before finding a comfortable position again. Should he wish to try an exercise routine to aid recovery, he should consult a qualified manual therapist. Occasionally a person is prescribed exercises that are not tailored to the individual; this can do more harm than good if the person holds any position that increases the pain.

Whether or not he should go back to work depends on the type of work he does, and what caused his back pain. A job involving a lot of sitting, for example, should be avoided in the case of a disc prolapse, and work involving heavy lifting or twisting should be avoided for as long as possible by any back pain sufferers.

Q I suffer from frequent, painful attacks of sciatica. Massage in the region of my lower back helps with the pain, but what can be done to prevent future attacks?

A Sciatica is not actually a diagnosis or a disorder, it has increasingly become a term that is used to refer to a shooting pain felt down one or both legs. To classically fit the description of sciatica, the pain should be in the distribution of the sciatic nerve. The sciatic nerve is made up of nerve roots that stem from the lumbosacral spine. It is the largest nerve in the body and travels down the back of the thigh, then splits to extend down the outside of the leg and back of the leg into the foot (see p31).

A variety of structures in the spine can cause pressure upon any or all of the nerve roots. This pressure creates the sensation of pain down the distribution of the sciatic nerve, which is why pressure on nerve roots at the level of the spine may be felt in the leg.

Regular neural mobility exercises (see p44) should substantially reduce occurrences of sciatic pain. Some individuals even benefit from yoga and Pilates; with any

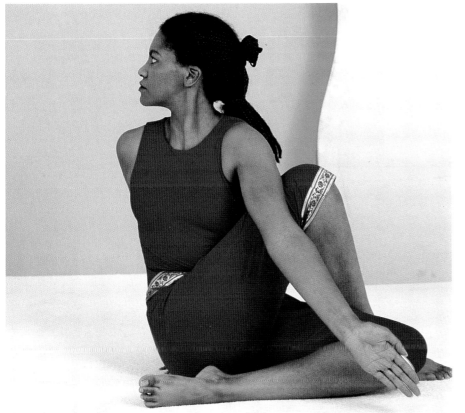

preventative measure the emphasis should be on getting into a routine of stretching and strengthening rather than sporadic episodes. This is where organized regular classes can be beneficial.

Heat and massage in the area of the lower back will relax the surrounding structures and release the tension around the nerve, but this will only provide temporary relief. In cases of extreme pain you should consult a qualified therapist who will be able to diagnose and treat your condition accordingly.

Q I was recently diagnosed with a prolapsed disc. Is my back now permanently damaged? Will I always have back problems as a result?

A The symptoms resulting from a prolapsed disc vary enormously and do not necessarily relate to the size of the disc prolapse. It is interesting to note that when painless backs are scanned many completely asymptomatic disc prolapses are discovered. This makes the diagnosis of a disc prolapse as the definitive cause of pain more complicated. It has been suggested that the symptoms probably relate to the speed at which the disc prolapse occurs.

It is difficult to predict how long symptoms will last. Some patients have extreme pain for six weeks without a recurrence while others have pain for a number of years. There are, however, a number of steps that should definitely be taken to improve your chances of a good recovery. First, you need to understand that the disc is put under the greatest pressure when you sit, lift and twist. Any activity during which the lower back is flexed (bent forward) will increase the pressure on the discs. These activities should be

stopped completely for the first three weeks of pain to allow the tissues to repair and to prevent further tearing. It is difficult to avoid sitting, but it is worth being strict with yourself and finding alternatives such as eating from a raised table, or lying on the floor while watching television. There are a number of ergonomic aids that are useful for reducing the amount of flexion in the lumber spine. These include cushions that reduce the amount your hips are flexed and that push into the small of your back allowing you to sit more upright (see p76). Lumbar support cushions can be attached to your office chair or car seat.

If lifting is unavoidable with your occupation, whether you have suffered from lower back pain or not, it is strongly advised that you receive lifting training from an ergonomist or physical therapist. They will teach you how to keep the object as close to your center of gravity as possible, with minimal twisting or flexing of the spine (see p82 for guidelines with regard to lifting).

Vibration can also contribute to disc degeneration; as a result driving or working with vibrating machinery can aggravate symptoms and reduce healing. After the acute stage it is important to seek an exercise program to strengthen the muscles that support the back.

Q I've heard that smoking can be a contributing factor to back pain. Is this true?

A Smoking is a well recognized risk factor for back pain, particularly intermittent back pain or pain that continues over a long period of time. One reason for this is that smoking causes blood vessels to constrict; this primarily affects the areas of the body relying on small blood vessels for their nutrition. The spine and outer parts of the intervertebral discs rely on small blood vessels for their nutrition. It has been argued that smoking reduces the blood supply and as such can contribute to the degenerative process.

Smoking is also associated with reduced levels of vitamin C. Vitamin C is essential for the health and repair of tissues and a reduction in the level of vitamin C contributes to degeneration and inflammation. If you are a smoker, it is recommended that you stop for these and a myriad other health reasons. If you find this difficult or impossible then a vitamin C supplement is advisable.

Q I'm 40 years old and I occasionally suffer from episodes of back pain. In addition to these instances my back is also increasingly stiff or more painful in the morning. Why is this?

A Pain in the morning can be due to inflammation, as well as the stretching of muscles and structures in your back that have been inactive for the whole night. Inflammation is the basic reaction of tissues to any injury; because there is less movement of the tissues overnight, there is less drainage of the injured area and this can cause a build-up of chemicals leading to swelling, which can compress nerve endings, causing pain.

The duration of pain in the mornings varies, depending on the amount of inflammation. Osteoarthritis typically causes between 10 minutes and half an hour of pain and stiffness in the morning, while rheumatoid arthritis and other more inflammatory conditions can cause up to two hours of increased pain in the mornings. If your pain in the morning does not ease for an hour or longer you should consult a manual therapist.

If your pain is not prolonged and not related to a medical condition, you should try a few exercises, such as the ones mentioned on pp34-39, to mobilize stiff structures and loosen muscles that may have been tensed due to previous injury.

Q My son has been diagnosed with Scheuermann's disease. What is this and can we do anything to combat the disease?

A Although a number of theories have been proposed, the cause of Scheuermann's disease is unknown. In most cases, the condition is diagnosed in the early teenage years and is usually detected by parents who are concerned about poor posture. The most common area for Scheuermann's disease is the thoracic spine, but it can also affect the lower back. Symptoms usually include the presence of an increased curve in the upper back (kyphosis), rounded shoulders and intermittent back pain. As the kyphosis increases, cartilage growing in front of the spine is placed under increased pressure, causing the growth of the cartilage to slow. Slow growth in the front of the spine coupled with faster growth in the back of the spine worsens the curvature.

Treatment of Scheuermann's is indicated to relieve pain, to correct an unacceptable cosmetic deformity and to prevent potential progression of the curve. An exercise program is recommended, together with the use of a brace, which can improve the curve during the growing years. Exercise alone is rarely of benefit, but may help to alleviate the element of back pain experienced when fatigue is present. (See Chapter 4 for strengthening and stretching exercises, in particular the scapula and hamstrings.)

GLOSSARY

Active system: refers to your muscle system, as opposed to the passive system which consists of ligaments and non-contractile fibers.

Acute pain: rapid onset of pain, as opposed to chronic pain that has been experienced for some time.

Annulus fibrosus: the ring-shaped, outer layer of the intervertebral disc.

Capsule: a fibrous structure that covers joints, helping with joint stability and supporting the synovial membrane which provides the joint fluid.

Cardiovascular: refers to the heart and networks of blood vessels. The cardiovascular system effects the circulation of blood through the body. Blood transports nutrients and oxygen to the tissues and helps with the removal of waste products.

Cartilage: dense, flexible connective tissue. During the early stages of human development the body contains many cartilaginous structures. Most of these soon disappear. In the adult, cartilage can still be found lining the joints and a few other structures of the body.

Central nervous system: nerve tissue of the brain and spinal cord that controls and coordinates the activities of the body.

Chronic pain: refers to ongoing pain as opposed to acute pain, which has a rapid onset.

Circulation system: see cardiovascular

Degeneration: the deterioration and loss of specialized functions of the cells of a tissue or organ. These organs can no longer perform their functions properly.

Digestive system: includes the mouth, stomach and small and large intestine. Food is digested and broken down into a form that can be absorbed and assimilated by the tissues of the body.

Disc (intervertebral disc): a round, relatively flat, flexible plate of fibro-cartilage that connects two adjacent vertebrae.

Disc prolapse: when the gel-like nucleus of the intervertebral disc (nucleus pulposus) ruptures, compromising the outer layer (annulus fibrosus) and in many cases leading to compression of a nerve and associated lower back pain.

Extension: the straightening or stretching of a joint; associated with backward bending of the vertebral column or spine.

Facet joint: a synovial articular joint that lies between two vertebrae. There are two pairs of facet joints in each intervertebral segment.

Fascia: connective tissue forming membranous layers of variable thickness through the body. Fascia surround the softer, more delicate organs and are divided into superficial fascia (found immediately beneath the skin) and deep fascia (forming sheaths that link to the muscles).

Femoral nerve: a nerve that extends down the thigh, supplying the quadriceps (muscles from the lower back extending to the front of the thigh) and the skin of the medial leg. The femoral nerve arises from the lumbar plexus.

Flexion: the bending of a joint from the anatomical position; movement associated with forward bending of the vertebral column or spine.

Flexor: the muscle that causes flexion.

Fusion: the fixing together of two structures, which usually renders them subsequently immobile.

Growth plate: a specific area at the top and bottom of a bone, including the vertebra where growth still takes place.

Hamstrings: a group of muscles at the back of the thigh. The hamstrings bend the knee and help move the leg backwards.

Hypermobile: excessive amount of movement.

Hypomobile: reduction of normal movement.

Immune system: a system in the body that produces antibodies, for protection against infection.

Inflammation: the body's response to acute or chronic injury. Involves pain, heat, redness, swelling and loss of function in the affected area. Blood vessels near the site of injury are dilated so that blood flow is increased locally to help with the healing process.

Intervertebral disc: *see* Disc.

Kyphosis: thoracic curvature of the spine.

Ligament: a tough band of white fibrous connective tissue that links two bones together usually close to a joint. Ligaments are non-elastic but flexible. They strengthen the joint and limit its range of movement.

Lordosis: cervical or lumbar curvature of the spine.

Lymph: the fluid in the lymphatic system. This fluid bathes the tissues, removing waste products which are eventually excreted from the body.

Manipulation: similar to mobilization but a more specialized movement. It is essential that the individual being manipulated remain relaxed during the manipulation process.

Mobilization: the movement of a patient by a practitioner to produce a desired therapeutic effect in a specific structure of the body.

Muscle: tissue that has the ability to contract, producing movement or force. The contraction of a muscle produces movement in a specific joint, for example, the knee or elbow.

Musculoskeletal: comprises both the flexible muscle system and the bony skeletal system.

Nerve endings: the final part of one of the branches of a nerve fiber. A nerve ending on the motor system is where the neuron either makes contact with another neuron at a synapse or with a muscle at a neuromuscular junction.

Nervous system: neural elements of the body, including the central nervous system.

Neural: refers to the nervous system.

Nucleus pulposus: a gel-like pliable structure; at the inner core of the intervertebral disc

Ossification: the formation of bone.

USEFUL ADDRESSES

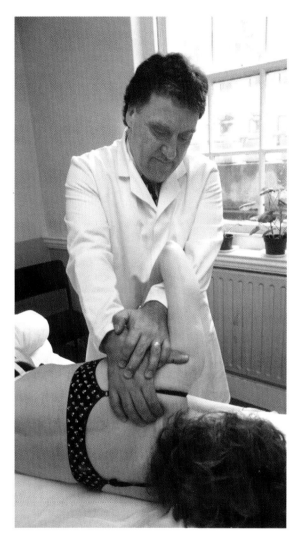

Toll-free Tel: 1-800-986-4636
Fax: (703) 243-2593
Website: www.amerchiro.org

World Federation of Chiropractic
3080 Yonge Street
Suite 5065
Toronto, Ontario
M4N 3N1
Tel: (416) 484-9978
Fax: (416) 484-9665
E-mail: info@wfc.org
Website: www.wfc.org

OSTEOPATHY
American Osteopathic Association
142 East Ontario Street
Chicago, Illinois
60611
Toll-free Tel: 1-800-621-1773
Tel: (312) 202-8000
Fax: (312) 202-8200
E-mail: info@aoa-net.org
Website: www.aoa-net.org

PHYSIOTHERAPY
Canadian Physiotherapy Association
2345 Yonge Street
Suite 410
Toronto, Ontario
M4P 2E5
Tel: (416) 932-1888
Toll-free Tel: 1-800-387-8679
Fax: (416) 932-9708
E-mail: information@physiotherapy.ca
Website: www.physiotherapy.ca

Alberta Physiotherapy Association
Suite 401 Energy Square
10109–106 Street
Edmonton, Alberta
T5J 3L7
Tel: (780) 431-0569
Toll-free Tel: 1-877-431-0569
Fax: (780) 431-1069
Website: www.albertaphysio.org

Physiotherapy Association of BC
1755 West Broadway
Suite 402
Vancouver, British Columbia
V6J 4S5
Tel: (604) 736-5130
Fax: (604) 736-5606
E-mail: pabc@bcphysio.org
Website: www.bcphysio.org

Ontario Physiotherapy Association
55 Eglinton Avenue East
Suite 210
Toronto, Ontario
M4P 1G8
Tel: (416) 322-6866
Fax: (416) 322-6705
Website: www.opa.on.ca

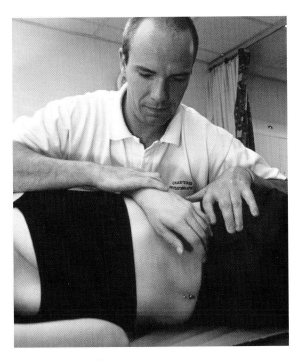

E-mail: physiomail@opa.on.ca

American Physical Therapy Association
1111 North Fairfax Street
Alexandria, Virginia
22314-1488
Tel: (703) 684- 2782
Toll-free Tel: 1-800-999-2782
TDD: (703) 683-6748
Fax: (703) 684-7343
Website: www.apta.org

OTHERS
The Rolf Institute of Structural Integration
205 Canyon Blvd.
Boulder, Colorado
80302
Toll-free Tel: 1-800-530-8875
Tel: (303) 449-5903
Fax: (303)449-5978
Website: www.rolf.org

Feldenkrais Guild of North America
3611 S.W. Hood Avenue
Suite 100
Portland, Oregon
97201
Toll-free Tel: 1-800-775-2118
Fax: (503) 221-6616

E-mail: guild@feldenkrais.com
Website: www.feldenkrais.com

Hellerwork International
3435 M Street
Eureka, California
95503
Toll-free Tel: 1-800-392-3900
Fax: (707) 441-4949
E-mail: hellerwork@hellerwork.com
Website: www.hellerwork.com

American Massage Therapy Association
820 Davis Street
Suite 100
Evanston, Illinois
60201
Toll-free Tel: 1-888-843-2682
Fax: 847-864-1178
E-mail: info@inet.amtamassage.org
Website: www.amtamassage.org

American Organization for Bodywork Therapies of Asia
1010 Haddonfield-Berlin Road
Suite 408
Voorhees, New Jersey
08043
Tel: (856) 782-1616
Fax: (856) 782-1653
E-mail: aobta@prodigy.net
Website: www.aobta.org

American Society for the Alexander Technique
P.O. Box 60008
Florence, Massachusetts
01062
Toll-free Tel: 1-800-473-0620
E-mail: alexandertech@earthlink.net
Website: www.alexandertech.com

American Holistic Medical Association
12101 Menaul Blvd. N.E.
Suite C
Albuquerque, New Mexico
87112
Tel: (505) 292-7788
Fax: (505) 293-7582
E-mail: info@holisticmedicine.org
Website: www.holisticmedicine.org

INDEX

PICTURE CREDITS

All photography by Ryno Reyneke, with the exception of those supplied by the following photographers and/or agencies (copyright rests with these individuals and/or their agencies):

Cover ....Photodisc/Gallo Images	93-94 ....Stone/Gallo Images
2-6 ....Stone/Gallo Images	97 ....The Image Bank
8-9 ....Ian Lansdale	98................t ....John Walmsley Photography
10-12 ....Stone/Gallo Images	98................b ....Photofusion Picture Library
13 ....Struik Image Library	99 ....Photofusion Picture Library
14-15 ....The Image Bank	100 ....British Chiropractic Association
16 ....John Birdsall Photography	101 ....Photofusion Picture Library
18-19 ....Stone/Gallo Images (Pty) Ltd	102-103....................Medipics/Dan McCoy
33 ....The Image Bank	104 ....John Walmsley Photography
78 ....Imagingbody.com	105 ....Wellcome Photo Library
85 ....Stone/Gallo Images	106-110 ....Struik Image Library
86 ....Stone/Gallo Images	111.............................Travel Ink/Colin Marshall
88 ....Stone/Gallo Images	113 ....Struik Image Library
90 ....Stone/Gallo Images	116-117 ....Struik Image Library

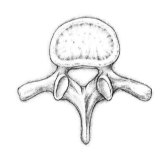

REFERENCES

Hutson, M. A. (1993) *Back Pain: Recognition and Management.* London. Butterworth Heinemann Ltd.

Porter (1982) *Management of Back Pain.* Edinburgh. Churchill Livingstone.

Porterfield, J. A. and De Rosa, C. (2nd edition, 1998) *Mechanical Low Back Pain.* USA. W. B. Saunders.

Twomey, L. T. and Taylor, J. R. (1994) *Physical Therapy of the Lower Back.* Churchill Livingstone.

Kendall, F. P. and McCreary, E. K. (1993) *Muscle Testing and Function.* Williams & Wilkins.

Petty, N. J and Moore, A. P. (1998) *Neuromusculoskeletal Examination and Assessment.* Churchill Livingstone.

Key, Sarah (2000) *Back Sufferer's Bible.* London. Vermilion/Random House.